ADHD ADDults

Your adventure to better health, wealth, success, and happiness begins now.

Think 'different'
Live 'different'
Do 'different'

DAVID JAMES (JIM) LIVINGSTONE

Copyright © 2022 David James (Jim) Livingstone

Published by: Absolute Author Publishing House

ISBN: 978-1-64953-543-6

All rights reserved. This book or any portion thereof may not be reproduced or used in any manner whatsoever without the express written permission of the publisher except for the use of brief quotations in a book review.

All images, logos, quotes, and trademarks included in this book are subject to use according to trademark and copyright laws in the United States of America

Disclaimer; Although this publication is designed to provide accurate information regarding the subject matter covered, the publisher and the author assume no responsibility for errors, inaccuracies, omissions, or any other inconsistencies herein.

This publication is meant as a source of valuable information for the reader. However, the author is not engaged in providing psychological, medical or other professional services. If expert assistance or counseling is needed, the services of a competent professional should be sought.

Library of Congress Control Number: 2022915872

Printed in The United States of America

Website: www.adhdaddults.com

Email: jim@adhdaddults.com

ALL RIGHTS RESERVED BY

David James (Jim) Livingstone

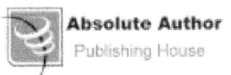

Content

Dedication	7
Acknowledgements	9
PREFACE	11
INTRODUCTION	15
1 - WHAT IS ADD/ADHD?	19
2 - MASTER YOUR ADHD MIND(S)	45
3 - YOUR GOALS AND SUCCESS	59
4 - YOUR BELIEFS AND SUCCESS	79
5 - WHY CHANGE YOUR BELIEFS?	97
6 - CHANGING YOUR BELIEFS	109
7 - YOUR BIG S.I.M.P.L.E. GOALS	119
8 - YOUR THOUGHTS	137
9 - YOUR EMOTIONS & FEELINGS	153
10 - YOUR BEHAVIOUR	167
11 - YOUR ACTIONS	183
12 - 7 KEY ELEMENTS FOR ACTION	193
13 - YOUR SUCCESS	223
CONCLUSION	229
References	235
ADHD ADDults Toolbox Index	237

Dedication

To the many with ADHD who fight their private, unseen battles and do extraordinary things on ordinary days.

For Louise, for believing in me.

Acknowledgements

To the many people who helps refine and improve this book with skills that were beyond my ability. My editors, Emma Moylan, Jessie Raymond and Michelle Balfour. Ben from Cascadia Author Services, Scribe School and Book Baby for their outstanding articles and encouragement. To Google and YouTube who supplied unlimited resources and information.

To my teachers and mentors past and present in no particular order.

Napoleon Hill, Joseph Murphy, Norman Vincent Peale, Prentice Mulford, Earl Nightingale, Charles F Haanel, Jim Rohn, Tony Robbins, Brian Tracy, Jack Canfield, John Assaraf, David Cameron Gikandi, T Harv Eker, Henry David Thoreau, Dale Carnegie, Bob Proctor, Shawn Achor, Steve Pavlina, Claude M Bristol, Stephen R Covey, John C Maxwell, Ken Robinson, Gary van Warmerdam, Dean Graziosi, Eckhart Tolle, Ronda Byrne, Dza Kilung Rinpoche, Peter Thiel, Dr Wayne Dyer, David A Greenwood, Dr Joe Dispenza, Robin Sharma, Richard J Leider, Brendan Burchard, Mike Bayer, Simon Sinek, Simon Foster, Ed Mylett, Gary Vaynerchuk, Wallace D Wattles, Deepak Chopra, Stuart Wilde, Daniel G Amen, Ari Tuckman, Martin Seligman, Dr Russell Barkley, Dr 'Ed' Hallowell, Douglas A. Puryear, Rachel Knight, Morty Lefkoe, Charles Duhigg, David Allen, Paul Orfale, Mark Manson, Peter Shankman, MJ DeMarco, Nir Eyal, Richard Koch, George Sachs, Gina Pera. Mel Robbins, James Clear, Thomas E Brown, Phil Boissiere, Tim Ferris, Susan C Pinsky

.

PREFACE

MY ADD STORY

ADHD/ADD is a subject I have a lot of experience with. I am seventy and was first diagnosed when I was forty-five.

I am grateful for getting some understanding of my failed relationships and catastrophic business failures.

I am also grateful for my fruitful relationships and the many highly successful businesses I started.

I was bored witless and struggled to learn at school. I was expelled in the last term of my final year of high school.

ADD or ADHD wasn't even a 'condition' when I was growing up. I was regularly described as overactive, a pain in the arse, bored, or stupid. I survived for forty-five years, not knowing that ADD existed until I was diagnosed with it in 1998.

Before my diagnosis, I self-medicated with alcohol, tobacco, fast cars, risky behaviour, and high-risk business ventures to get the dopamine that was missing from my brain. I had also developed some seriously limiting and defective beliefs about myself and life in general.

After I managed to destroy a marriage, my relationship with my daughter, and several successful businesses, I started looking for solutions by first getting sober, which I did at age thirty-six.

Getting sober was the right decision for me. However, initially, it made dealing with ADD more challenging. I had no escape at the end of the day; I couldn't stop the constant negative chatter in my mind.

Sobriety did not solve my problems; they just became more visible and inescapable. I had to face them head-on. I became a self-development junkie.

At age sixty-five, I finally took my ADD seriously after I managed to undo twenty years of work by starting a business I was passionate about but knew nothing about. The thrill of starting from scratch was too powerful for me to resist.

I had to get my dopamine and adrenaline from the massive risk and challenges of something new beyond my current abilities. I was ON the whole time.

That I could fail never entered my head; my executive function was on an extended holiday. After three years of massive effort to create a healthy carbonated protein drink – *Xrcise Fuel* – we lost everything and had to borrow money from family and friends to survive.

I was on and off medication during this time, never taking my ADD/ADHD seriously.

Looking back, I can connect the dots, which explains why I did the things I did that made my life and the lives of those around me more difficult than they needed to be.

I was ill-equipped to accept, understand and manage my ADD, and many of the professionals I sought help from didn't specialise in adult ADD. I couldn't utilise all the self-development information I had spent the last twenty-five years studying.

Starting from scratch was going to be a challenge. I was repeating the same behaviours, and I had to find out why.

I have spent the last four years working through my history to understand the significant issues holding me back.

PREFACE

This book is the result and will guide you in recognising, understanding and using your ADHD abilities, so you can lead an exciting, productive and rich life while avoiding the unnecessary pain and frustration I have experienced.

The person I am today wants to thank the person I was for refusing to give up.

'If you're going through hell, keep going.'

Winston Churchill

INTRODUCTION

Different is not a disorder.

Your unique ADD/ADHD individuality means you learn and use information in a different way. You are built the same but wired differently.

Traditional neurotypical methods won't work. You need a unique path and process.

ADHD doesn't discriminate and affects millions of people of all levels of intelligence and from all walks of life. Welcome aboard the ADHD Express.

- Do you feel like you don't fit in … anywhere?
- Are you struggling to know where to start, what to do and when to do it?
- Does your mind spin with all the possibilities until physical and psychological chaos takes over?
- Are you struggling to keep your head above water, overwhelmed by the constant stress caused by impulsivity, procrastination and disorganisation?
- Do you feel overwhelmed by too much information, distractions or stimuli?

- Do you feel like you'll never be able to get your life under control or fulfil your potential?
- Do you experience low self-esteem and a sense of insecurity?
- Are you constantly changing your mind or looking for new stimulating challenges? (**S**hiny **o**bject **s**yndrome.)

First, learn how to manage, then master, your ADHD mind and go from just surviving to thriving. Not despite your ADHD but because of it.

NEUROTYPICAL INFORMATION IS THE PROBLEM

The Internet has provided unlimited resources, with an explosion of information and misinformation. Your mental evolution can't keep pace with the knowledge overload.

While the marketing and promotion of personal development have exploded with technology, the basics remain the same. I believe the hype has overtaken the content.

Your ADHD brain is trying to navigate through a self-development minefield designed by and for neurotypical minds.

Almost all resources on self-improvement were not written for neurodivergent ADHD minds. Which only leads to confusion, feeling overwhelmed, and paralysis.

My goal is to provide you with ADHD-friendly self-development in a simplified, structured format.

With this in mind, I was careful to get straight to the point when writing. Exercises in this book are intentionally made short to eliminate your excuse of 'not having enough time' and to stop you from getting bored or distracted.

While science backs up everything I've written, this book is not an academic or medical research paper; it's a users' guide, a concise summary.

INTRODUCTION

I was diagnosed with ADD in my forties, about thirty years ago, and have been on and off medication (dexamfetamine) ever since.

While learning, accepting and studying ADHD, I have tried and tested many strategies with great successes and catastrophic failures.

I want to help other ADHDers cut through the bullsh*t and avoid the frustration and pain I went through. These are not theories; they are time-proven structures and strategies that work in the ADHD world.

UNLOCK YOUR UNIQUE ADHD/ADD TALENTS

> '*I cannot teach you anything;*
> *I can only encourage you to think ...*'
>
> **Socrates**

You need a guide, not a 'guru'. No expert is smarter or better than you; they have *learned* to become experts. Their desire to grow and time in the game is what makes them the experts.

You must become an expert on yourself. To unlock your unique abilities and embrace your ADHD traits, you need to understand how *your* ADHD mind works.

YOUR BEST LIFE

> *You can't outsource your own self-development.*

Personal improvement is in your DNA, and you are capable of leading an exciting, fulfilling and extraordinary life.

ADHD ADDults

There's nothing wrong with where you are right now. You are wired to seek constant improvement, to make your life better. Better has no final destination, and better does not mean perfect.

There are no secrets. Every book written on self-development (including this one) can be traced back to documents and books written hundreds or thousands of years ago and updated in various forms.

There are no magic keys or steps to transform your mind and life overnight. But if you are prepared to do the work, there are proven techniques and effective pathways.

A ROAD MAP TO YOUR SUCCESS

The right books, videos and knowledge can change your life, but only if you study them with the clear intention to learn and take immediate action to implement what you have learned.

Each of the following chapters has been structured in a particular format and sequence that builds the foundations for you to experience a full life, your best life using your ADHD strengths.

Only you have the power to act on your life and affect the outcome. Find your place in this amazing world by being different and using your ADHD to your advantage.

But, first, you need a basic understanding of how your ADHD mind works, so let's get started.

To your health, wealth and happiness!

> 'Go confidently in the direction of your dreams! Live the life you've imagined.'
>
> **Henry David Thoreau**

1

WHAT IS ADD/ADHD?

*ADHD is not a disability.
It's a different ability.*

ADHD is essentially a chemical issue in the management systems of the brain. It is not a lack of willpower, laziness or being away with the fairies. The difficulties you've experienced stem from ADHD – they are not a result of personal weakness or a character flaw.

Neuroimaging studies show that ADHD [1] is caused by structural and chemical variations in the brain responsible for the essential roles of focus, motivation, attention and behaviour.

ADHD is not a behaviour disorder, nor is it not a mental illness or a specific learning disability. ADHD is, instead, a developmental impairment of the brain's self-management system.

ADHD ADDults

This research highlights what individuals with ADHD already know. It can be challenging to know what to do, where to start and when to do it.(2).

You can spin in all the possibilities until physical and psychological chaos takes over. Feelings of dissatisfaction and frustration in your inner world are then substantiated by events in your outer world.

This is because you have not fully developed your ability to engage the most valuable part of your brain, the prefrontal cortex (PFC).

It is like having a new 75-inch smart TV with incredible surround sound, superb picture quality and a vast range of channels and options, but you don't have any batteries for the remote.

There's nothing wrong with the TV. It's just that the signal impulses aren't getting to the black box. You're excited and happy with the new TV but frustrated because you can't use the benefits you know it has.

Imagine you're running late for your plane and the only way to get to the departure gate is going <u>up</u> the <u>down</u> escalator with your laptop, cabin bag and two small children. You might make it, but you'll be exhausted and aggravate a lot of people getting there.

YOUR ADHD ABILITIES

Your ADHD package comes with some unique talents.

- *Empathy* – the ability to sense other people's emotions and imagine what someone else might be thinking or feeling.

WHAT IS ADD/ADHD?

- *Ingenuity* – your ability to solve problems, often with clever, original and inventive ideas.
- *Enthusiasm* – you bring intense enjoyment and excitement to life.
- *Hyper-focus* – your capacity to hyper-focus is something that you can use to your benefit. When focused on a specific goal or target, it can be an unbelievable positive feature that helps you succeed.
- *Light-hearted* – you love to laugh and make others laugh as well.
- *Spirit* – you can bounce back from challenges.
- *Intuition* – you have the power of acute observation and deduction and a sharp sense of awareness.
- *Creativity* – ADHDers produce some of the world's best ideas. Your ability to generate multiple solutions to challenges is something that most people miss.
- *Unrelenting curiosity* – the more interested and committed you are in your life, the greater your chances of success. Curiosity is behind everything discovered, built and brought into existence you see around you.
- *Cool in a crisis* – You can think clearly in life-threatening situations.

Learn to capitalise on your different skills and talents. Your perceived greatest weakness can be your greatest gift. Be inspired by the novelty of change. Utilise your faster processing speed to your advantage. Embrace your ADHD; own it. Wrap it around you like body armour. Use it for all it's worth every day.

It is who you are and what makes you great.

Instead of trying to be perfect, you need to accept your limitations and make sure that you don't let what you cannot do interfere with what you can do.

> *'It is far more lucrative to leverage your strengths, instead of attempting to fix all the chinks in your armor.'*
>
> **Tim Ferriss**

Many adults with ADHD, such as Olympic swimmer Michael Phelps; British celebrity chef Jamie Oliver; Virgin Airlines founder, Sir Richard Branson; lead singer of Maroon 5 and vocal coach on the popular TV show *The Voice*, Adam Levine; and Grammy award-winning artist will.i.am, have found meaningful ways to manage their traits, take advantage of their talents, and lead productive and satisfying lives.

> *'If someone told me I could be normal or continue to have ADD, I would take the ADD.'*
>
> **David Neeleman, Jet Blue Airways founder**

DIRECT YOUR ATTENTION

> *'Individuals with ADHD do not have a deficit of attention; they have an abundance of attention. The challenge is controlling it.'*
>
> **Ned Hallowell, MD, and John Ratey, MD**

Learn to use your attention. You have the remarkable ability to pay attention, focus and even hyper-focus on things that interest you.

You also can disregard things that don't interest you. You have high levels of energy and outside-the-box thinking. You have drive and enthusiasm.

You are optimistic and excel at pushing past setbacks, adopting new strategies and moving forward.

You are bright, creative and funny, willing to take risks and be spontaneous.

You can see a different and unique perspective on situations that others cannot.

The positives far outweigh the negatives. You need to learn to play to your strengths, modify your lifestyle, think constructively, meditate, and build structure and rituals into your daily life, including the weekends.

We will go into the how-to for achieving this in later chapters.

For now, acknowledge the challenges and benefits of ADHD and learn to compensate for any boring bits you must perform in pursuit of your higher objectives.

If you feel that you don't fit into this world, *that's great* because you are meant to help create a different and better world. Don't make the mistake of trying hard to fit in. Instead, work on what makes you stand out.

> *'If you're lucky enough to be different,*
> *don't ever change.'*
>
> **Taylor Swift**

CHALLENGES

Don't use ADHD as an excuse. It's an explanation.

Just as we have duality, positive and negative, up and down, north and south, night and day, high and low tide, ADHD does have some challenges along with its benefits. You may have a few or many of these; it doesn't matter. You are not defined by them.

- You might have trouble staying motivated to do the boring bits that are a part of daily life. ADHD doesn't discriminate and affects people of all levels of intelligence and from all walks of life.
- You may tend to be disorganised, procrastinate, experience trouble starting and finishing projects, and underestimate the time it will take to complete tasks. You can be hypersensitive to criticism and hyperactive mentally and/or physically.
- You could be easily distracted by low-priority activities or external events that others tend to ignore or have so many simultaneous thoughts that it's difficult to follow just one. You may feel like you'll never be able to get your life under control or fulfil your potential.
- You may experience low self-esteem and a sense of insecurity or underachievement. You may feel like you've been struggling to keep your head above water or are overwhelmed by the constant stress of procrastination, disorganisation and handling demands at the last minute.
- You may experience career difficulties and feel a strong sense of underachievement, affecting your work, relationships and self-confidence.
- Taking on too many projects simultaneously can be an issue. As can the constant desire for high stimulation, a low threshold for boredom and a dislike of established channels.

- Hyperactivity, impulsivity and inattentive behaviour are natural, innate tendencies rather than wilful, self-determined actions.
- ADHD can contribute to various health problems, including compulsive eating, substance abuse, anxiety, chronic stress, and tension.
- Research shows that defiance is a common attribute of ADHD, where people directly defy authority as an automatic position. ADHDers are also often very prepared to argue their case against authority, rather than going along with something that they think is wrong. (19)
- You have high aspirations and energy and are creative, but daily performance can be a bit erratic, and consistency is challenging. You want to be successful, but some days your old behaviours and habits short circuit your potential.

Many people have spent years seeing what they should be doing but falling short. And that experience, quite directly, undermines this aspect of the motivation – as they continually fail to achieve goals, they lose faith in themselves. However, this is not your destiny. You can be successful if you set your mind to it.

> *'I didn't let ADHD prevent me from achieving my goals, and neither should you.'*
>
> **Howie Mandel**

YOUR ADHD MIND AND SUCCESS

People often associate ADHD with the trait's adverse effects, which is inaccurate and limited thinking on the issue. It is more like an attribute with some powerful positive benefits. Like all traits, it must be understood and managed to get the best from it.

We make people nervous because we don't play by their rules, which for them creates uncertainty and fear. They prefer for us to stay within the white lines and not make waves.

The three main characteristics that many professionals believe determine if you have ADHD are a great example of a traditional limited mindset versus a growth mindset. Seeing the glass half empty instead of seeing it half full.

- They say distractibility – I think unrelenting curiosity.
- They say impulsivity – I think unlimited creativity.
- They say hyperactivity – I think high energy.

VICTIM OR VICTORIOUS?

Dump the bullsh*t ADHD disability story you have been fed and are still reading and posting about. Yes, you have challenges, but you must focus on the positive benefits ADHD provides. You can't think about your ADHD in any negative way because your brain can only hold a negative or a positive thought. If you are still predominately thinking limiting thoughts about your ADHD, you can't fully exploit your positive skills and abilities.

ADHD is about grabbing hold of an idea that you're excited about and channelling all your energy into that. With that mindset it's amazing what you can achieve.

YOUR MIND

> 'You have power over your mind – not outside events. Realize this, and you will find strength.'
>
> **Marcus Aurelius**

Nothing is more critical than unlocking and using your mind's creative power. It might help eliminate famine, sickness, global warming, and wars. It can provide abundance for everyone and allow people to share their unique talents and joy with this world.

The brain is an organ, but the mind isn't. The brain is the physical place where the mind lives. Your brain coordinates your movements and your activities and transmits impulses. But you use your mind to think. You can reflect on what happened, and what may happen.

Your conscious mind combines thought, perception, emotion, determination, memory and imagination within the brain. The mind provides the awareness of conscious thoughts and the ability to control what you do and understand why you are doing it.

UNDERSTAND YOUR MIND

You need to devote time to getting to know how your mind works. Call it mindfulness, meditation or quiet solo time. Time spent understanding your mind is just as important as that spent eating and exercising.

When you try focusing your mind on breathing or trees and flowers when you walk in nature, what does your mind do? It wanders all over the place – mostly bringing up ANTs (automatic negative thoughts) or unsolved problems.

If left unchecked, it can take you out of the peacefulness of the present moment and into a downward spiral.

If you don't want to keep making the same mistakes, learn from your past experiences. Strengthen your mental control by becoming aware of your thoughts and focusing on the positive thoughts you want to have.

You become what you think about.

YOUR ADHD BRAIN

The brain is approximately 2 per cent of your body weight and uses over 20 per cent of your energy.

Neuroscience reveals that neuroplasticity is your brain's ability to change its structure and function in response to outside stimuli and internal activity.

If you have a thought and experience an emotion, it's because your brain has done something ... handing out droplets of neurochemicals.

NEUROCHEMICALS

Dopamine – the missing link.

ADHDers generally have a dopamine shortage.[3] That is why you may seek out dopamine and adrenaline-producing careers, activities or sports to compensate for the lower flow rate of dopamine your brain experiences.

The challenge with these activities is that you may indulge in behaviour risky to your physical, financial, emotional and relationship health.

Dopamine has been called the pleasure molecule, the reward chemical that makes you feel good.[4] Many studies show that your brain adjusts to the dopamine hit from a repeated pattern by reducing the flow and impact.

That is why, as you get used to a new activity, new relationship, new clothes or a new car, some of the excitement and pleasure goes out of the experience. It is more like a novelty reward chemical – your brain responds more to new experiences than repeated patterns.

You continually look for ways to get your natural chemical cocktail. This explains your desire for change and distraction. Your ADD brain is easily bored and always searching for the next bright shiny object. You are looking for more novelty and excitement. It's looking for a natural chemical hit!

The challenge lies in finding positive, non-destructive pathways to achieve it. You have high energy, and when you can't find a suitable outlet, you can shut down, just like the crash of a computer, leaving you feeling empty and flat.

You need to channel your enthusiasm and energy to positively unleash your drive and creativity.

Let's use the fictitious Dave, as an example. Dave's *dopamine fix* comes from skydiving. This is when his mind is clearest. He is removed from emails, mobile phones, and trivia. His only responsibility is opening his chute, and that makes life simple.

Individuals with ADHD display fewer symptoms in novel or unfamiliar surroundings or when tasks are more unusual and exciting.

Example

First responders like firefighters, police and emergency personnel get their fix from the intensity and laser focus of the situation.

Research shows you can use physical activity to increase your dopamine, adrenaline and serotonin levels. Something as quick as doing ten push-ups, air squats or running a couple of flights of stairs is enough to chemically 'charge' your brain. The dopamine and serotonin your brain produces will help you refocus.

Curiosity, novelty and change will also trigger a dopamine release.(20)

DOPAMINE REWARDS

You must also develop the ability to tap into your dopamine reward system while pursuing your goals. Link rewards to milestones and the effort or action taken, not just the final achievement. Start with simple small steps that allow you to build up to your major goals.

Devise internal and external sources of motivation and rewards to keep the dopamine flowing. Motivation is temporary and serves its purpose. Your drive is what will keep you going when inspiration takes a holiday. It comes from your *why* – your reason for being here, your purpose, which you can discover in later chapters.

YOUR ENVIRONMENT

Armed with an understanding of your ADHD challenges, you can make real changes in your life. To get the best from your life, develop your organisational skills for your life, home, office, desk and car. Remove the mess and clutter from inside your head and your environment.

You have to put your talents and skills to work in the right environment where you can thrive. Your environment plays a massive part in your life.

- Physical – the state of your body
- Mental – the condition of your mind
- Career – your career or business choices
- Home – your family or significant other
- Relationships – your social network
- Financial – thriving over surviving
- Contribution – a reason for breathing

ADHDers must keep busy, or depression shows up.

When you have ADHD, part of energy management is planning your day and creating an environment where you can do the essential things you need to get done.

Figure out your strengths and set up your environment in a way that supports them. Also, work out your weaknesses and remove them either temporarily or permanently from your environment.

> **Example**
>
> *I used to have lots of stuff on my computer screen. I put all the files into one huge file that I open to get out only want I need to work on, which helps keep me from getting distracted.*
>
> *I still write lots of notes on paper. They all go into the bottom drawer of my desk; out of sight is out of mind. At the end of each month, I go through the drawer, throw out what isn't relevant, act on the critical few, and dump the trivial many.*

Create boundaries for yourself and others, set the stage for your day and life, and be selectively available. Practise triage … can't do it all? Try to pick the most important single task. Remove all distractions.

Clarity and focus are the cornerstones of your success. Don't overcommit or have too many obligations. Practise saying no. Start saying no to your dog, if you must, but get comfortable with saying no. If you can't say no, say let me think about it. Many times, the request will disappear.

Your mental environment is one aspect essential to your health, wealth and happiness, over which you have full control. Ask yourself what work environment would make the most of your ADHD strengths?

STRUCTURE

It is remarkable how much simpler your world becomes with an organised internal balance. Structure offers you support, reducing your ability to self-destruct through procrastination or by giving up.

For any project to be done efficiently, it needs a flexible structure with a beginning, a middle and an end. It also needs to be prioritised with set timelines. This will help prevent you from feeling challenged by the size and scope of any project.

Structure is essential to your success and happiness. It's the world you create for yourself. It gives you control over your environment, reducing your tendency to self-sabotage through distractions, impulsivity and procrastination.

You may struggle to organise and regulate the behaviour needed to accomplish your long-term goals. Structure provides the support and the links in the chain to help you achieve your goals.

Achieving goals requires you to plan, start and finish tasks, stay organised, handle frustration, recall and follow multi-step directions, stay on track, self-monitor, and change what isn't working.

You may find it challenging to stay on target and frequently change your mind because of the shiny object syndrome. Like a butterfly, you float from idea to idea. This can have a very limiting or disempowering effect on you.

Your ADHD mind can struggle with starting and finishing projects in a time and energy-effective manner because you don't know where to start.

So, you either don't start or you jump into the middle of a task and work in different directions, leading to confusion and frustration.

One of the keys to your success is building an external structure that is creatively loose but demands challenge. If you perceive it as too

You are what you repeatedly do and become what you continually think about. Over long periods, your thinking patterns become etched into the billions of neurons in your brain, connecting them in unique, entrenched ways.

When specific brain pathways connected between different components or ideas are frequently repeated, the neurons begin to 'fire' or transmit information together in a rapid, interconnected sequence. Once the first thought starts, the whole series gets activated.

You must learn to master your mind. You need to listen, get to know your mind, acknowledge its contribution, understand its nature, implement a retraining program, and treat it kindly.

EXECUTIVE FUNCTION

Many of your behaviours occur without conscious thought, like breathing or stepping out of the way of an oncoming car. However, to plan, monitor and successfully execute your goals, you rely on the executive function part of your brain.

Executive function (EF) describes a set of mental processes and skills that help you live a full, successful and happy life. Any process or goal pursuit that requires time and energy management, decision-making, and storing information in one's memory uses your executive function to varying degrees.

EF provides the mental abilities you need to regulate your behaviour towards the present and future and engage in goal-directed actions.

Think of executive function as your project manager (PM), whose sole purpose is to help you reach your full potential and achieve your dreams and goals.

Some of the tasks your project manager needs to do to make your life enjoyable and fulfilling are.

- Clarifying your major life goals

WHAT IS ADD/ADHD?

invasive, you will feel trapped. However, you still need to be tethered to reality. Structure and rituals provide that stability.

ENERGY MANAGEMENT AND TIME LOSS

You can't change time. It is like gravity, and it's the same for everyone – twenty-four-hour days. To reach your goals, you must manage your energy within each twenty-four-hour window of opportunity.

Time is your most valuable resource and can't be recovered, so invest it, don't waste it. (See Chapter 12.)

Each day you need:

- Physical energy to work and play
- Emotional energy to connect
- Mental energy to learn and grow
- Spiritual energy to contribute

Fatigue and time of the day can impact ADHD symptom severity. Everyone is different – some people thrive as early birds, while others are better suited to being night owls. Work out what is best for you and do your most challenging tasks when your energy levels are their highest.

Match your energy to the task. It is difficult to make good decisions when you are mentally, emotionally or physically tired.

AWARENESS

This involves noticing where your mind goes when it wanders and gently bringing it back to the focus on breathing, eating, walking, loving or working. When you do this repeatedly over months or years, you begin to rewire and retrain your brain.

Over time you begin to know when your mind is checked out or spinning its wheels, and you can gently guide it to get back on task. When it tries to take off on its own, you can gently remind it that it's an interdependent and essential part of the whole of you.

WHAT IS ADD/ADHD?

- Targeted focus
- Goal setting, planning and the ability to see your future
- Staying on course and adjusting to unforeseen challenges
- Goal achievement
- Decision-making
- Self-discipline
- Setting priorities
- Effective time and energy use
- Managing thoughts and prioritising activities in a logical sequence
- Controlling emotional responses
- Delaying gratification to reach your long-term goals
- Defeating procrastination
- Remembering all the aspects and details of a job
- Problem-solving, perceiving, sensing time and managing your energy
- Setting micro dopamine reward milestones

Your project manager is very busy and needs these skills and abilities to help YOU succeed.

- Self-awareness
- Self-discipline
- Vision
- Thought management
- Emotional management
- Self-motivation
- Planning and problem-solving skills

Your ADHD challenge is to develop these abilities to understand and effectively use your brain's executive function capabilities to manage your behaviour to set and achieve your life's goals.

Living and working in the proper physical and mental environments is vital for your PM to operate effectively and efficiently.

PREFRONTAL CORTEX – YOUR HR DEPARTMENT

The prefrontal cortex (PFC) part of your brain provides the resources to help your project manager focus, analyse thoughts, pay attention, learn, concentrate on goals and regulate behaviour.(5)

This includes mediating conflicting thoughts, making choices between right and wrong, and predicting the probable outcomes of actions or events. This area of your brain makes short-term and long-term decisions.

Your ADHD PFC can be a bit of a loose cannon or be out to lunch when you need it most. There are no traffic lights or stop signs controlling which messages get through.

You are more likely to react to whatever is holding your attention at that moment – the current message and emotion, leading to some potentially dangerous conditions ahead.

EMOTIONAL CONTROL

Emotions run through the intersection of the PFC,(6) bringing quick mood changes. Impulsive worry, anger, sadness or excitement seem to come from nowhere when the emotion is an immediate reaction to an event that just occurred.

You may be more sensitive than others to rejection, teasing, criticism or your perception that you have failed or fallen short. This is the definition of a condition called rejection-sensitive dysphoria (RSD), which is common among people with ADHD.(18)

What is dominating your thoughts at that moment is responsible for the emotions and feelings you are experiencing. Therefore, you may express feelings more intensely than may be justified for a given situation.

LIMITED WORKING MEMORY

ADHDers have a limited memory capacity.(7) However, there are ways around this obstacle. You have the creative ability to come up with different methods of building a solid working memory system.

> **Example**
>
> *Because my working memory is sh*t, I don't retain important information, great ideas, passwords or anything I learn. I used to waste a lot of time going over the same stuff.*
>
> *I designed an external visual working memory using multiple PowerPoint presentations. One for each major area of my life. This helps prevent me from getting distracted by one area or another as I used to when they were all on a single seventy-seven-page presentation.*
>
> *I like colour and visuals, so most of the slides are covered in images that snap my mind back to the strategies, ideas, goals and dreams that are important to me. I don't have to try and rethink all the important points. It saves me a lot of time and frustration, and it reminds me why I am doing what I am doing.*
>
> *I also put brief, to-the-point notes at the bottom of the slides to help prevent distractions. This provides all of the important, relevant information all in one area. Really important sh*t I print out just in case the backup systems fail or my laptop dies.*
>
> *A printed version also allows me to take it somewhere quiet and away from my normal working environment to review or get a different perspective on things.*

BEHAVIOUR/IMPULSIVITY

You see countless unique possibilities, all competing for and winning your attention. You are often told you have such potential but never seem to make progress.

Your natural inclination is to focus on what interests you the most and ignore those areas that don't capture your attention. But sometimes, this trait can result in harmful procrastination and have unwanted outcomes.

Your impulsive actions can work for or against you. They bring you pleasure and success or pain and loss.

In the following chapters, you will learn to gain greater control over your actions and reactions.

ADDICTION

Adults with ADHD tend to self-medicate or spend too much money on unnecessary items, looking for quick gratification instead of more significant, sustainable long-term rewards.

Stimulant medications are very good at keeping your brain from getting distracted once it is engaged, but you are still 100 per cent responsible for getting your mind engaged in the first place.

Addiction comes in many forms, including social media, money, work, alcohol, drugs, sex, overthinking, bright shiny objects, and you can add your own.

Your brain is seeking dopamine. You have to find healthy ways to provide it that are beneficial to you with limited risk and downside. Finding balance is your challenge.

SELF-DISCIPLINE

ADHD can affect your self-discipline and hinder your ability to see your long-term goals, create effective strategies, take the necessary actions to achieve them, and stay on course long enough to reach your goals.

You must find a way to spark interest in transforming tedious tasks using your creativity and imagination. You have passionate thoughts and emotions that are more intense than those of the average person. The mental quest for dopamine can drive you through incredibly tricky circumstances.

THINKING

To thrive, you must develop your ability to control and direct your thinking; it is vital to your happiness and success.

Thinking is necessary for sustained goal setting and persistence. These are the actual mental abilities required to solve problems, persist when something gets tricky, and target long-term goals by establishing realistic steps and following through to success.

Even with a healthy mindset and discipline, ADHD can cause you to drift away from your plans. You know what you should be doing or hope to accomplish, but not how to make that happen.

As you go through this book, I will provide you with some possible 'how-to' ideas and options.

You are trying so hard, repeatedly, and still not achieving your goals or meeting social expectations. These failures make you think negatively about yourself, leading to low self-esteem, which impacts your motivation.

You can learn to master your mind and thoughts rather than letting them master you.

HYPER-FOCUS

One bonus of this skill is it allows you to get a lot done. It can also be used to defeat distraction – a way of tuning out the chaos. It can be so strong that you become oblivious to everything happening around you.

Use your hyper-focus abilities to your advantage and channel them into productive activities.

On the downside, this can also lead to work and relationship problems if left unchecked. Finding a way to stop paying attention can be as important as learning to direct your attention.

Set up schedules, time blocks, breaks and barriers to prevent you from crashing through the STOP signs.

CONNECTION

The importance of connecting with your like-minded community, your tribe, can't be underestimated. Psychologists from Maslow to Baumeister have repeatedly stressed that a sense of connection is one of your fundamental human needs.

First, connect with yourself. You must know who you are and have confidence in yourself if you desire to connect with others. If you don't believe in who you are and where you want to go, work on that before doing anything else.

Human beings are inherently social creatures. Social groups provide us with an essential part of our identity, and more than that, they teach us a set of skills that help us live our lives. Feeling connected, especially in an increasingly isolated world, is more critical than ever.

Social isolation is an incorrect term; physical isolation is the issue. Physical isolation is a complete or near-complete lack of contact between an individual and society.

FACE TO FACE

Research indicates that we likely benefit more from increasing face-to-face physical interaction. (8) Instead of retreating into your phones' perceived comfort, you need to put down your devices and engage with those in the world around you. Connect with the barista making your morning coffee and talk to the supermarket cashier.

Strong ties with family, friends and your community provide you with happiness, security, support and a sense of purpose. Being connected and engaged with others is vital for your mental and physical well-being and can be a protective factor against stress and worry.

Loneliness is a feeling of a lack of companionship or quality relationships with other people. Changes in your circumstances and lifestyle can result in feeling less connected to others.

However, loneliness is not an inevitable part of life – there are many things you can do to expand and strengthen your social networks.

If you want to be closer to others in your existing relationships, you can improve your communication and emotional connections.

Equally, if you'd like to meet new people and form meaningful friendships, there are many opportunities to join groups or connect one-to-one with people who share your interests and personal values.

Organisations worldwide offer social programs and services specifically for ADHD individuals, catering to people of all ages.

ALTERNATIVE OPTIONS

If the symptoms of ADHD are still getting in the way of your life, despite self-help efforts to manage them, it may be time to seek outside support. Adults with ADHD can benefit from several treatments, including behavioural coaching, individual therapy, self-help groups, vocational counselling, ADHD coaching, educational assistance, and medication.

ADHD treatment works best when designed to suit an individual's brain, not clusters of textbook symptoms; the same applies to your self-development.

My intention is that you not only enjoy some social time but also receive information from quality sources and health professionals while supporting and being supported by other members.

☺

*I tried being normal once.
The most boring two minutes of my life!*

SUMMARY

- You are *not* broken.
- Different is *not* a disorder.
- Note the challenges but focus on the positives.
- Don't try to fit in; exploit what makes you different.
- ADHD is not a lack of willpower, personal weakness, or flawed character. It's a chemical issue.

Accept that managing your ADHD isn't about curing it. It's about awareness of when you aren't where you want to be ... and knowing how to get back.

It's a never-ending process. Sure, it will get easier with time, practice and patience. But you will make mistakes. Everybody does. Learn and move on.

ACTIONS

1. Start by accepting your ADHD brain has provided you with some unique and amazing abilities mixed with a few challenges to help you grow. Focus on knowing and using your strengths and managing your challenges. Look for different, creative solutions for both. Write down 3–5 examples of each and schedule a time to start taking action.

2. Create your ADHD-friendly environment, both at work and home. Tidy up your car, home, and work areas. Set boundaries for yourself and others, set the stage for your day and your life, be selectively available.
3. Reward yourself with quality dopamine activities beneficial to you and the planet. Try some form of exercise, listen to music, learn something new, read something inspiring, go for a walk in nature, a drive in the country, whatever works for you. Do something new or different once a week.
4. Prioritise. You can't do it all at once; narrow your options down, then select your single most important task, set a time block, remove all other distractions, and hyper-focus until the timer goes off. Repeat.
5. Practice mental and physical self-care. Feed your mind and body with quality nutritional food, cut out the crap. Get a massage. Grab ten minutes of quiet solo time each day and build the ritual. Practice being grateful for what you have while pursuing what you want.

> 'Life's challenges are not supposed to paralyze you, they're supposed to help you discover who you are.'
>
> **Bernice Johnson Reagon**

Please remember you are not alone. ADHD impacts millions. Connect at **www.adhdaddults.com** for ADHD support

NOTES

2

MASTER YOUR ADHD MIND(S)

Mastery of your thoughts and feelings is your highest possible achievement.

YOUR CONSCIOUS MIND

Your conscious mind is like a computer screen. It is a focusing tool, not a storage place. It has no memory. It can deal with only one thought at a time, positive or negative, 'yes' or 'no'.

You can learn to choose and change your thoughts.

Take your ADHD, for instance. You have two choices. One is to blame your ADHD. *I have a mental disorder, a neurological imbalance in my brain, and therefore I am doomed to fail.*

Or you can focus on the positive traits of your ADHD. *I have some very special talents, and therefore I am sure to succeed.*

You get to choose.

- The conscious mind receives information from your five senses. It is logical, rational, inquisitive, personal, emotional and selective.
- It is home to your thoughts, hopes and desires.
- Your awareness of yourself and the world around you is part of your consciousness.
- The conscious mind has a very limited capacity compared to your subconscious mind. However, your conscious mind can influence some of the automatic programs running in your subconscious.

The role of the conscious mind is only to choose the goal. The path to the goal is prepared by the subconscious mind.

Because your ADHD mind is always on the move and fails to retain information, you must constantly feed it positive thoughts and affirmations. Thus, you must learn to control the thoughts you hold in your conscious mind so you can instruct your subconscious mind. Initially, it may not be easy, but it is possible and gets easier and faster with practice.

> *In pursuit of your goals, if your conscious mind does not give new and different instructions, your subconscious mind will do nothing different and no change will occur. Tomorrow will be a repeat of today.*

Using your conscious mind, you can choose your new thoughts and ideas and turn them into images and feelings conveyed to the subconscious mind and alter the course of your life.

THE SUBCONSCIOUS MIND

> *'If you think you can, or if you think you can't, either way, you're right.'*
>
> **Henry Ford**

Your subconscious mind controls over 90 per cent of your life. You live your life based on how your subconscious mind was programmed in the past.

It is the silent creator of your life and will bring all that you feel and believe to be true into the physical world.

The subconscious mind is subjective, illogical, impersonal, neutral, and can't distinguish between real and imaginary, nor does it care. It simply responds according to the positive or negative thoughts you consistently hold in your conscious mind.

- Your subconscious mind loves imagery, simple words, and feelings.
- It speaks to you in intuitions, impulses, hunches, urges and ideas. Your subconscious will respond to the vibrations of your strongest conscious thoughts.
- It starts the actions needed to achieve the results that align perfectly with the information you provided and is the source of power and the cause of every effect or outcome in your life. It drives all your conscious actions that lead to your results.
- The subconscious is open to suggestions from the conscious mind. The subconscious always accepts as true that which you feel to be true.

Throughout life, your brain retains the ability to change its structure and function in response to your experiences.(9)

Your subconscious mind never fails to deliver that which has been impressed upon it by your conscious mind.

That thoughts become things is a universal law.

The subconscious mind never alters the accepted beliefs you consciously hold. It is affected by repetition, intensity and your current thoughts. Whatever is currently 'top of mind'.

Your subconscious mind is extremely powerful and is the gateway to living the life of your dreams. Later chapters will show you 'how to' manage and master your subconscious mind.

MANAGE YOUR SUBCONSCIOUS

Your subconscious is the link between your conscious mind and the infinite intelligence of the superconscious mind.

It is very easy to live as you already have because you can just let your unconscious mind do the work. However, this is not ideal if you want to change your life.

By leaving your life to your subconscious mind, it will maintain the status quo and your life will not change. You have to raise your level of awareness and make conscious changes in the present moment.

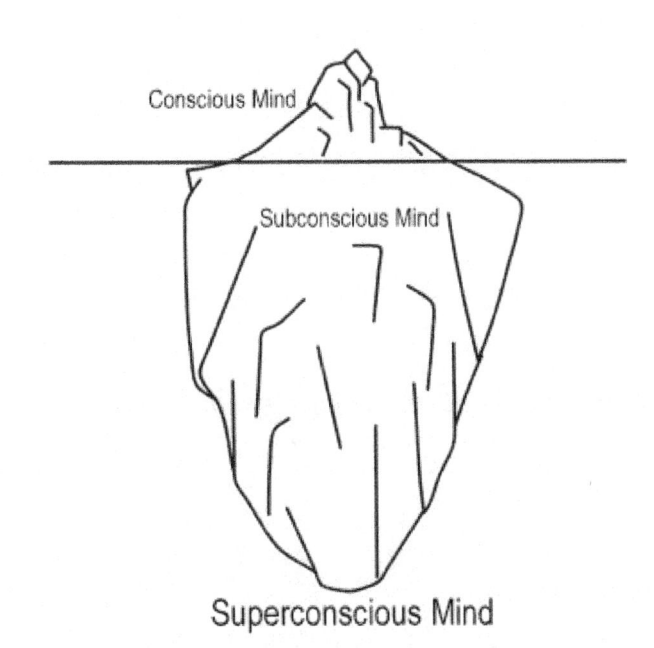

Conscious Mind

Subconscious Mind

Superconscious Mind

The subconscious does not originate ideas but accepts those that your conscious mind feels to be true. It can't differentiate between what is real or imagined, nor does it care.

Ideas are impressed upon the subconscious mind through images and feelings. No concept can be accepted by the subconscious until it is felt.

To impress the subconscious with your desired outcome, you must use your imagination to create the feelings you would experience as having already achieved your clear and specific result.

EXAMPLE

Imagine you are standing in the home of your dreams or driving your dream car along a winding mountain pass. Feel the sheer joy and excitement of the moment. With practice, you can build very intense feelings in your mind and body.

This is a powerful way to convey your desires to your subconscious mind that will now start working on ways to deliver that exact experience to you as quickly as possible.

Sleep and meditation are the pathways that bridge the gap between the conscious and the very powerful and dominant subconscious. They are the best ways to impress your desires and goals into the subconscious, which accepts as true that which you feel as true.

Through your ability to think, feel and change, you have dominion over your life.

Create a calm state, visualise what you desire to achieve in life, and feel the desire fulfilled.

As the desired result is accepted, become indifferent to possible failure, for acceptance of the end provides the means to that end.

You don't need to know how the end is achieved. Be secure in the knowledge that the outcome has been perfectly defined and the means will unfold.

The moment you accept that your desire is a done deal, your subconscious finds the means for its manifestation.

Images and feelings are the means through which your desires are conveyed to your subconscious.

IMAGES

Vision is by far our most dominant sense, taking up half of our brain's resources. Visual processing doesn't just assist in the perception of our world. It dominates our worldview. Visual processing takes up about half of everything your brain does.

Imagery is the most effective way to communicate with and program your subconscious. Hear a piece of information, and three days later, you'll remember 10 per cent of it. Add a picture, and you'll remember 65 per cent.

Pictures beat text, in part because reading is so inefficient for us. Our brain sees words as lots of tiny pictures, and we have to identify certain features in the letters to be able to read them. That takes time.

Why is vision such a big deal to us? Perhaps because it's how we've always apprehended major threats, food supplies, and reproductive opportunities.(10)

> **Example**
>
> *Visual images work best for me, so I put together a series of PowerPoint slides with powerful images with selected text that provide my brain with dopamine and feel the corresponding uplifting emotions.*
>
> *To avoid my brain getting bored and not producing dopamine, I have built up a library of different slides for the same goal so I can vary the images, and my brain thinks it's new and lets a few drops of dopamine flow.*

Use powerful visual images of your goals and dreams fuelled by your strong feelings for their attainment to pull you through when motivation and willpower take a holiday.

See yourself doing the necessary small tasks along the way to reach your goals.

Everything is created twice, first in your imagination, then in the physical world.

MEDITATION – SOLO TIME

> *'The mind is definitely something that can be transformed, and meditation is a means to transform it.'*
>
> **14th Dalai Lama**

Schedule daily solo time, free from distractions and the 'noise' of everyday life. Experiment with time – I would suggest starting with ten minutes and seeing how it goes. Commitment and consistency are vital. Develop the process into a ritual.

Use this time to do your creative thinking, not to problem solve.

The purpose of meditation is to open the pathway between your conscious, subconscious and superconscious (infinite intelligence), which already holds all the answers and solutions you need to achieve your goals and dreams.

Meditation has the following benefits.(17)

- Makes your ADHD mind work better and increases your concentration.
- Improves physical, mental and emotional health.
- You sleep more deeply and have more energy.
- Reduces stress and anxiety.
- Raises your level of self-awareness.

Meditation is training your mind and cultivating awareness, thereby giving you greater control over your energy, thoughts and emotions.

To meditate successfully, picture and feel your goals and dreams as already fulfilled. Feel the emotion as if all your goals and dreams have already been achieved.

Ideally, create a passive state, similar to the reflective and relaxed feelings that precede sleep.

Meditation calms the senses to the outer world and makes your mind open to suggestions from within. It primarily helps you reach a tranquil state and enables you to connect with your higher power (whatever you conceive that to be).

Forms of meditation vary. It can be done by sitting in a comfortable chair, lying on a bed or the floor, walking outside or running.

How, when and where to meditate is only limited by your imagination, not your circumstances. Do what works for you. I suggest you try a couple of different types. While the process is important, it's the results you are after.

Never meditate or go to sleep feeling discouraged or dissatisfied. Clear your mind of any real or imaginary problems, fears or doubts, and completely detach your mind from the day's events.

Let your thoughts flow through your mind like leaves on a stream. Try taking yourself to a relaxed and serene place in your mind. It could be sitting on an isolated beach, walking through a forest or whatever appeals to you.

Take time to meditate every day.

SUMMARY

- Your subconscious mind never rests.
- Success is mastering your subconscious mind.
- Use your conscious mind to influence and direct your subconscious mind.

MASTER YOUR ADHD MIND(S)

- Sleep and meditation are the links to your powerful subconscious mind.
- Trust your subconscious to provide the answers and solutions you are seeking.

ACTIONS

1. Practice awareness – start monitoring your thoughts during the day. Who's in control?
2. Are you running on auto or making conscious decisions? Set your mobile alarm 3–4 times a day, and when it goes off, stop and think briefly about how you are feeling and the beliefs and thoughts behind the feelings.
3. Write down the positive thoughts you want your conscious mind to use to influence your subconscious mind and repeat them throughout the day.
4. Make the subconscious mind your biggest supporter. Let go of being confined to the known and step into the unknown, and you can transform your life.
5. Start meditating for 5 to 10 minutes each day to calm your mind and tap into your powerful subconscious mind without concerns about the results; just start.
6. Stop confusing your subconscious mind by constantly changing your conscious mind. Start disciplining your mind to stay on task. Take control of what you decide to think about. When you notice your mind wandering, bring your focus back to the task at hand.
7. Meditation is a process and it takes some time to feel natural and become a ritual you look forward to doing, but the benefits are huge.

BONUS EXERCISE … best done at night

7 STEPS TO ACCESS YOUR SUBCONSCIOUS

1. Release any tension and thoughts of your day. Relax your body and calm your mind with deep breathing. Clear your

mind of any real or imaginary problems, any fears or doubt, and completely detach your mind from the day's events.
2. Get your request over to your subconscious mind. What solution or advice are you seeking? Select only one issue at a time and put one simple, clear question to the subconscious. Write it on paper for clarity.
3. Ask for creative solutions or ideas that benefit you and all concerned. Your subconscious speaks to you in intuitions, impulses, hunches, urges and ideas.
4. Receive – be open to the messages from your subconscious. This may take some trial and error to interrupt the feedback you receive properly, but it gets easier with practice. You will get to a point where you know it is what you are seeking.
5. Now feel like you would when you have your solution. Then relax and quietly drop off to sleep.
6. On receiving an answer or solution, write it down immediately, express gratitude for receiving it, and take some form of immediate action.
7. Repeat each night.

All the answers and solutions you seek are available to your subconscious mind. Ask without doubt or fear with the confidence that the answers will appear from the superconscious mind.

You have to attach yourself to a wisdom and a power that transcends your understanding, like the wind, you can't see it, but you can feel its effect.

Trust your subconscious.

NOTES

3

YOUR GOALS AND SUCCESS

For ADHDers, goals are not about money, cars, houses, position or relationships. It is the emotions, the feeling you are seeking. It's about brain chemistry.

☺

Live your life by design, not by default.

Goals are the stepping stones to your dreams. The pathway to reach your objectives and fulfil your purpose. A goal is an idea of the future or the desired result.

Many people today are sleepwalking through life. Even though they work hard, they don't feel like they are getting what they want. That's because they don't know what they want; there is no clear vision of success.

When you stop to set goals and think about what you want, you break out of autopilot and start designing a life by conscious choice. Be proactive, take charge and think about what you want for yourself.

Setting and achieving your goals helps you live your life in alignment with your values, needs and dreams. When you do that, you have so much more to give to your family and friends, your career and the universe.

Your goals give you direction and help you develop a mind map as to where to invest your time, resources and energy.

It helps you focus on acquiring specific knowledge and skills and organise your time and your resources to make the most of your abilities.

Goals provide a solid framework that will help your ADHD brain use its formable power to hyper-focus on the things you deliberately choose to bring into your life. They give you long-term vision and short-term motivation.

Chapter 7 will help you set and achieve your dreams and goals.

YOUR WHY

To stay locked and loaded on your goals will be one of your biggest challenges. You need compelling reasons to help you go the distance.

You deserve to decide for yourself exactly what and who you'll become and what you'll experience and acquire in your life.

Are you driven more by curiosity, exploration and discovery – and less by competition and winning? You can still achieve what success means to you.

*There are many paths to the mountain top
but the view is still the same.*

Start examining your goals through the lens of *why*.

Why is this goal important to me? Ask yourself why you love it and why it's important in your life.

Determining why you want to achieve your goals helps you prioritise what is important to you and where you want to spend your precious time and energy.

Goal setting is not only about choosing the rewards you want to enjoy but also determining and accepting the sacrifices required to achieve your goal.

There are no right or wrong goals, just different ones; don't get hung up on what other people are doing. Your success and fulfilment will come from having the courage to live life on your terms.

You were built to conquer challenges, solve problems and achieve goals. Without obstacles to conquer and goals to achieve, there can be no real satisfaction or joy in life.

Attaining any goal requires you to go through a process. If you compromise the process by cutting corners, you're missing out on what goal achievement is about: personal growth through making the journey.

> *'The ultimate reason for setting goals is to entice you to become the person it takes to achieve them ...'*
>
> **Jim Rohn**

YOUR MISSION

> *'The purpose of life is to contribute in some way to make things better.'*
>
> **Robert F. Kennedy**

You have a vital role to play in the never-ending universal evolution of life and creation that has been going on since day one.

As with everyone before and everyone after you, we all contribute to the massive, never-ending evolution of the universe. We are all interconnected in this universal matrix.

We lack the knowledge and understanding of the complexities of our existence. You were given the amazing gift of life and the ability to think. Now is a good time to repay these gifts by living up to your potential in any field or endeavour you choose.

Have you already figured out the purpose of your life, the reason you are here? If not, as is the case for most of us, your goals and values can help answer this all-encompassing question. Think about it; knowing what you value gets you closer to an answer.

You have to identify what is important to know what you want to get and give in life. Your mission may change throughout your life as you gain experience and knowledge.

Your purpose may be exactly what you are doing now. Setting your goals aligned with your values gives insight into your purpose.

YOUR GOALS AND SUCCESS

Awareness and reflection help you adjust and set new goals and directions as you grow and pursue your life's mission. It is refined and discovered through your life experiences.

Your purpose is to reach your full potential by using your unique ADHD skills and talents every day in whatever you are doing and taking action in alignment with your goals and values.

You don't need to completely overhaul your life as you get more clarity about your mission; just lean into it, bit by bit.

Start living your mission a little more every day and pay attention to the feedback you're receiving from others, the results you are producing and how you are feeling.

Entrepreneur and investor Sam Altman says some of the best advice he ever received was, 'If you can't figure out what kind of work you like, pay attention to what's easy to concentrate on and gives you energy vs. what makes you tune out and feel tired'.

> *'If you haven't found it yet, keep looking …'*
>
> **Steve Jobs**

CLARITY

Clarity of purpose can be elusive and may change throughout your life. If you don't have clarity, then your attempts to focus on tasks, install new beliefs and more efficient habits, and release old habits will only fizzle.

It is like telling the Uber driver – I want to go to a restaurant for dinner. Great, they know you are hungry and don't want to cook at home. The rest is anyone's guess.

ADHD ADDults

Would you drive aimlessly through the city until you spot a restaurant that appeals to you? Hopefully not, yet that is how most people treat their life goals.

Ask, 'What exactly is it that I'm trying to accomplish here?' What gives you your greatest feeling of value and contribution? What accomplishments give you your deepest sense of achievement and satisfaction?

You must know your destination. Your specific written goals are the road map that provides clarity for your mind to work with.

They must be so clear that it would be possible for a stranger to look at your situation objectively and give you a straight 'yes' or 'no' response as to whether you've accomplished each goal.

Lack of clarity is the enemy of success.

YOUR VALUES

Values help clear out the clutter. People are consumed with so much these days. Identifying your values enables you to weed out the time and energy-wasting people and things from your life!

Living by your values builds your self-respect and acts as an anchor in turbulent times. It guides your behaviour and provides you with your code of conduct, your internal compass, your North Star.

There are no right or wrong values because we are all different by design. Your values should reflect what is important to you. Some values and their priority may change throughout your life.

Study your major goals, and you will see they reflect your deepest values. There may be a prominent theme that keeps reappearing that shows you the hierarchy of your values.

> **Example**
>
> *One of my major goals is to become the best version of myself through self-evolution. My mental and physical health become one of my top values to achieve this goal.*
>
> *I want optimum energy, vitality and physical health so I can experience life in all its lessons and blessings and contribute to the best of my ability.*
>
> *My ADHD brain thrives on the proven path of exercise and optimum nutrition and turns to sh*t if I fall off the wagon, which I still do from time to time.*

You will be more motivated to commit to and achieve goals aligned with your values, so you will be happier if you live a life based on your values.

You have general and core values. Most of your general, lower-level values have been influenced by your environment and upbringing. Your core values are locked in your DNA, embedded in every atom of your body and brain. Your own unique data dot code.

Whether you are aware of them and live by these values is another matter. Your core values may be buried under a mountain of superficial social, cultural and bullsh*t media values.

CORE VALUES

Your core values are what you value most in life.

You may not be aware of your core values or understand their level of importance in your life. When you live by your core values, you experience higher self-confidence and fulfilment.

Awareness of your core values helps you judge a situation when faced with multiple choices.

How do you determine your core values? Discover your core values through solitude and quiet time, and allow your goals and values to rise to the top. Try a walk in nature or solo time in a corner of your home, free from distractions.

Defining your values takes effort and is another step in knowing yourself. What gives you a sense of fulfilment in your life? Being creative? Going on adventures? Learning new things?

Below is a list of some core values. Use this list to start brainstorming the values that matter most to you. This list is by no means definitive. Feel free to add your own.

Abundance, accomplishment, achievement, adventure, altruism, approval, assertiveness, beauty, belonging, boldness, calmness, certainty, change, closeness, commitment, compassion, composure, contribution, control, determination, discipline, empathy, energy, equality, entertainment, enthusiasm, fairness, growth, harmony, health, independence, individuality, inspiration, integrity, love, meaning, nonconformity, openness, patience, passion, peace, prosperity, security, self-respect, success, status, trust, wealth, wisdom.

Choose five to eight core values from your list. Your unique core values won't define your individuality if you have too few. However, if you have too many, you won't put the amount of focus on any of them that is needed to leverage your personal growth.

Make sure that your values feel personal and unique to your identity. This may take several goes before you feel confident.

Pick the value that is the most important to you and go down your list. Once you have prioritised your list, wait a few days, and look at your list again. See if you still feel like you have listed your core values in the right order; take some time to move them around.

You may have competing values.

Example

Let's say one of your core values is achievement or financial success, and another is health and vitality. Your financial success cannot come at the expense of your health. You must avoid conflict between your values.

You may have to temporarily rearrange the priority of your core values to achieve your goals. If your number one core value is your health, but financially you are struggling, you can elevate your financial goals to the number one position until you get some stability in your finances.

Instead of exercising for thirty minutes six days a week, you could change that to twenty minutes three to four days a week, lift the energy of the workout, and adjust your nutrition accordingly. Use the saved time to invest in your finances.

You might value self-discipline yet struggle with discipline in some areas of your life; welcome aboard. You are in great company. Does that mean you should remove that value? Hell, no, it simply means you have some work to do. You are looking for progress, not perfection.

It's one thing to define your core values; the challenge is to live by them each day. Come up with a single sentence description of what that value looks like for you.

Example

Progress – I am always learning and evolving mentally, emotionally, financially and spiritually.

Health – Intelligent nutrition, regular exercise and eight hours of sleep are the foundations for my energy and success.

Simplicity – I seek the disciplined pursuit of simplicity and strive for the vital few, not the trivial many.

DEFINE YOUR SUCCESS

Success is making a positive difference in someone's life.

What is success? It is different for each person. Before you can set your goals, you have to get clear on what success means for you. How will you know you have achieved it? You cannot hit a target you cannot see.

Step away from society's expectations and start focusing on and refining your expectations. Suspend your current beliefs and personal judgment, and be free to choose goals that matter most to you.

Fortunately, your ADHD brain is blessed with great imagination and creativity. To set your goals, you need to use your imagination to create a clear picture of what success means to you and what your ideal life would look like.

Imagine the feelings associated with having already achieved your goal and see how deeply it affects you. This will help you gauge its importance.

YOUR IMAGINATION

> *'Imagination is more important than knowledge. It is the preview for life's coming attractions.'*
>
> **Albert Einstein**

Everything is created twice: first in the mind, then in the physical world.

Use your imagination to create pictures of your life's coming attractions. Imagination stimulates creativity and innovation.

You have an amazing gift to think outside the box. Allow your imagination the freedom to grow and evolve, which may create products or services that change the way you live.

Imagination is the key ingredient to expansion and the advancement of your life. Imagination is the ability to form a picture of something in your mind.

Your mind can build mental pictures of objects or events that currently do not exist. Every day, we use our imagination unknowingly for both positive and negative purposes.

You can imagine a series of events unfolding in your mind that may be false. Your imagination is a powerful resource that needs to be directed positively and productively.

Everything human beings have created started life in someone's imagination. Imagination is the way to unlock hidden doors and solve problems. Your imagination is the engine of your thoughts. It converts your thoughts into mental images. Learn to use this powerful resource to make your life better.

You need a controlled imagination with well-sustained thoughts firmly and repeatedly focused on your chosen goals. Stop your imagination from wandering off to areas that have no bearing on your desired outcomes.

Imagination is a much stronger force than willpower. Imagination will pull you towards your goals.

What you steadily focus your imagination on is what you attract.

YOUR VISION

Learn to use your imagination to visualise your ideal life in the present moment – bring your pictures to life as if you are watching a movie, and indulge all your senses. You are the lead character and the director.

When you use your imagination, you must focus on what you want, not what you don't want. Focus on the positives, like the benefits of

YOUR GOALS AND SUCCESS

great health and high energy, not on having to give up your favourite muffin or chocolate bar. Visualise wealth and abundance.

As you learn to use your imagination, always see your intended outcome in the present moment during your visualisation sessions. Imagine yourself being, doing and having that which you want to experience. This is a critical step when learning to use your imagination.

By consciously imagining the mental picture in the present moment, you are imprinting and programming your subconscious mind, which is where everything must first be created before it can appear in the physical realm. In contrast, by keeping your images in the future, your choices will stay there, in the future, and just out of reach.

The subconscious mind works best with images and emotions. Instead of imagining static pictures in your mind, try turning them into a movie. See yourself experiencing and enjoying a new career or loving relationship, perfect health, abundance or anything else.

Creative visualisation requires that you keep your thoughts focused on your specific outcome.

Do not become frustrated if your thoughts wander during the creative visualisation process. Simply relax, continue to breathe deeply, and bring your thoughts back to your intended outcome.

If you find that you cannot concentrate your thoughts, then bring yourself out of your relaxed state and come back to your visualisation session later.

This is a vital and learnable skill. It takes consistent practice to master any new process. Take it slowly, and do not try to force anything. Over time, your images will become clearer and sharper.

YOUR CREATIVITY

While imagination deals with 'unreal' thoughts that are free from the confines of reality, creativity is the means that brings imagination into the physical world.

Creativity is the practical process of doing something meaningful with your imagination. It is where the work starts. To be creative, you must take action.

As humans, it's in your DNA for you to want to create something and then, when that's created, move on to the next thing. Your ADHD brain wants change and novelty more often than most other people; getting the balance right is the challenge.

Your ADHD brain can play a huge part in providing creative solutions. You need your imagination and creativity to work together to create the life you want.

First, use your imagination to develop mental pictures of the life you want, then use your creativity to set and achieve goals to help you achieve it.

Instead of just coming from a linear, logical approach, your ADHD creative side can approach a situation from all angles, helping you see things differently and deal with uncertainty.

There is no right or wrong way to be creative. When you create, it allows you to engage with the world without judging yourself.

Being creative means taking calculated risks, ignoring doubt and facing fears. It means breaking with routine and doing something different to improve something. It could be your health, finances or other areas of your life.

It improves the way something is done to make it better, easier or adds additional value. You can be creative with social media or even how you make a coffee; the possibilities are endless.

Being creative means solving a problem in a new way. It means changing your perspective. You don't have to create the next big thing; just create a better experience for yourself and others.

Use your creativity to find solutions that move you towards your vision, dreams and goals.

DESIRE

Without desire, there is no goal.

Desire is the motivating force of life itself. It brings progress to the world and is the foundation of all achievements.

Desire is the super-charger that drives all human action. Without an intense desire, you will eventually give up on your dream no matter how hard you work.

The strength of the desire also determines the speed of manifestation. Weak desires equal weak results. To achieve any significant goal, you must have a burning desire to reach that goal.

Your desire must be cultivated, watered, and protected against weeds and ANTs (automatic negative thoughts). Sometimes, it is strong and thriving. Other times, it looks a little unloved.

Strong desire is the mental nutrition that feeds your mind.

You need to review your goals every day and take some form of action towards their achievement. It is the nutrients, the life-sustaining water for your garden of desire. If you stop watering, it will eventually wither and die.

Successful people do this, consciously or subconsciously. By taking consistent action each day, you stop the weeds of doubt from creeping in.

You were born with a desire to contribute and do something unique and meaningful with your life.

It may be to bring another precious life into this world, build homes for families, paint, write, explore, challenge traditional thinking, or anything deeply important to you.

Your desires and purpose are unique to you, as are your natural talents and ability to adapt and learn.

Ensure that you can't imagine your life without pursuing those goals that are meaningful to you. This is imperative; if you don't think of your goal as a necessity in your life and an absolute must, you won't achieve it.

BURNING DESIRE

Burning desire borders on being an obsession or addiction.

I believe most people are obsessed or addicted to some form of behaviour. You get to choose whether it's beneficial to yourself and the world! So why not be a little addicted or obsessed with the desires that benefit you, others and the planet.

ADHDers need to be aware of their attraction to new bright shiny objects and trends. Stay locked and loaded on your true heart's desires and purpose.

Desires and goals are essential for maintaining your sense of purpose and direction in a constantly changing world.

DECISIONS

> *The perceived benefit of indecision is that you cannot fail. You can live forever in the endless possibilities of your creative ADHD mind. The sad reality is you will never achieve anything.*

Setting goals requires making decisions, which can be a challenge for your ADHD mind. So many choices, so little time. What if I choose the wrong goals? What if I fail? What if something better comes up? What if ...?

Setting goals and achieving them takes commitment, but the rewards far outweigh the effort. Invest the time in yourself because you are capable and worthy.

With so many options, you might decide not to make a decision just yet ... and that develops into a habit that continues for years, for some people the rest of their lives. They spend their life undecided – which is chronic procrastination.

The universe is waiting on you, not the other way around, and it's going to keep waiting until you finally decide and select the goals and life you want. Life is about progress, not perfection.

Decisions are about choices and taking 'responsibility' for your choices. The challenge is that making a decision, even if it is the right decision, means you have to say no to other possibilities. Now that is something your ADHD mind dislikes.

Example

It's embarrassing to admit how many hours I used to waste trying to make decisions. The smallest, simplest things drained away all of my energy and time. After hours, days or weeks of careful deliberation, I would finally make a decision.

Then for no apparent reason, I would just do something completely different. It was mental torture. I was never at peace. I could never trust myself not to change my mind. Choices were my ultimate rabbit hole. Decisions became an exhausting bottomless pit.

> *I used to love allowing my creative mind to devise countless opportunities to pursue with my life. I could feel the excitement, the adrenaline rush of making lots of money as I built various businesses in my mind.*
>
> *I had all the lifestyle goals I wanted without ever having to do the hard yards to achieve them. Success was guaranteed; decisions had no consequences because I didn't have to make any.*
>
> *It was a very comfortable place to live. Unfortunately, it stopped me from evolving and taking action towards achieving my many goals and dreams. I spent more time living in my head than living in reality.*
>
> *I found that the marketplace only rewards you for the products or services you actually bring to the world, not what you daydream about providing ... bugger.*

Decision-making is a key skill you can and must develop to succeed in life. It is a major task of executive function that you can learn by putting structure and templates in place to guide you through the process.

This is covered in much greater detail in Chapter 12.

SUMMARY

- Live your life by design, not by default.
- Clarity is the bullseye to achievement.
- Define what 'success' looks like to you.
- A burning desire is vital to your success.
- Your primary mission is to evolve, learn, grow and enjoy life. To contribute and make the world better by putting your unique ADHD skills and talents to work.

YOUR GOALS AND SUCCESS

ACTIONS

Before you drive into settings your goals, which is covered in Chapter 7, you need to get clarity about what 'success' looks like for you, based on your values and purpose, your life's mission.

1. Delete any disempowering beliefs, thoughts, fears or doubts about your ability to be who you want to be, do what you want to do and have what you want to have.
2. Dump the past. Start with a clean slate and choose your top 10 values. Next, pick your top 5 values, then number them in priority.
3. Look for clues to your purpose by answering these questions.

   - Who inspires you? *Write a list.*
   - What excites you about this beautiful world? *Come up with your top 3 answers.*
   - What type of books, magazines, social media, and videos do you watch? What is the attraction? *Write it in a single word, like exciting, inspiring ...*
   - Now list the values you see in the above examples. Do they match your top values? If not, take a break, then redo these exercises.

What would you do if you were guaranteed to succeed? Don't worry about how. Dump all excuses, doubts and fears. *Write a private declaration of your purpose in a joyful and heartfelt sentence.* My example, I am constantly amazed and fascinated by ADHD people who do extraordinary things against all the odds, and I want to share their inspiring stories with the world.

Based on your values and purpose declaration, develop a clear picture of what success looks and feels like for you. *Capture your images and thoughts in a journal, mobile or PowerPoint presentation, and take 10 minutes to review them every day.*

NOTES

4

YOUR BELIEFS AND SUCCESS

> *'In any project, the essential factor is your belief. Without belief, there can be no successful outcome.'*
>
> **William James, philosopher and psychologist**

Think about that statement for a moment. Why do over 90 per cent of people who spend time, energy and money going to seminars, reading books, listening to podcasts and watching YouTube videos fail to permanently improve their lives in any substantial way?

They all received the same information, directions, tactics and strategies from the same teacher in the same format. Yet still, they fail to achieve their goals and dreams.

It is because even the best advice, knowledge and intentions can't overcome your limiting beliefs.

WHAT IS A BELIEF?

My reference to belief or faith is not from a religious perspective. Beliefs and faith are not the same things. Belief is a creation of your mind; faith is a creation of your spirit.

Beliefs have become shrouded in mystery, and it's time to remove the veil. Beliefs are just a resource, a tool to help you shape your life.

A belief is the result of you consciously or unconsciously giving meaning to events in your life.

They are patterns and habits of your mind, road maps that continually take you to the same destinations.

Your ADHD mind becomes addicted to these habits and is reluctant to change them, even though they may be damaging and unsupportive of your goals and dreams.

Still, beliefs are the foundations for all great achievements.

In their most basic form, your beliefs are the rules you have adopted for yourself that determine how you live your life.

A belief acts as a guiding principle for your behaviour and underpins your personal philosophy.

Your beliefs can generate strong emotions and behaviours. They can hold you back or propel you forward. Like GPS, your beliefs become your personal positioning system.

They are thoughts or ideas that you believe to be true. Your belief is your perception of the way things are, but this does not mean that your belief is true. Many beliefs are accepted as true without proof.

You were born with zero beliefs. You absorb them from your surroundings, from your family, friends, teachers and experiences throughout your life; you seldom question your beliefs.

Your rules support your belief structure and, therefore, your view of 'reality' and the identity you accept of yourself. They become embedded in your subconscious mind through repetition over time. You aren't consciously aware of most of the beliefs that drive your behaviours.

A belief reflects your 'map of the world'. Therefore, every thought you have, every decision you make, and your actions reflect a conscious or unconscious belief.

> *If you want to change your life, it starts with changing your beliefs.*

WHY YOUR BELIEFS MATTER

Life can be seen in many ways. It can be viewed as an adventure or as a struggle. The choice is always yours.

Life becomes an adventure when lived in the spirit of exploration and experimentation, rather than just as a survival contest. Be spontaneous, open and flexible with your beliefs and identity, which will provide you with positive energy and thoughts.

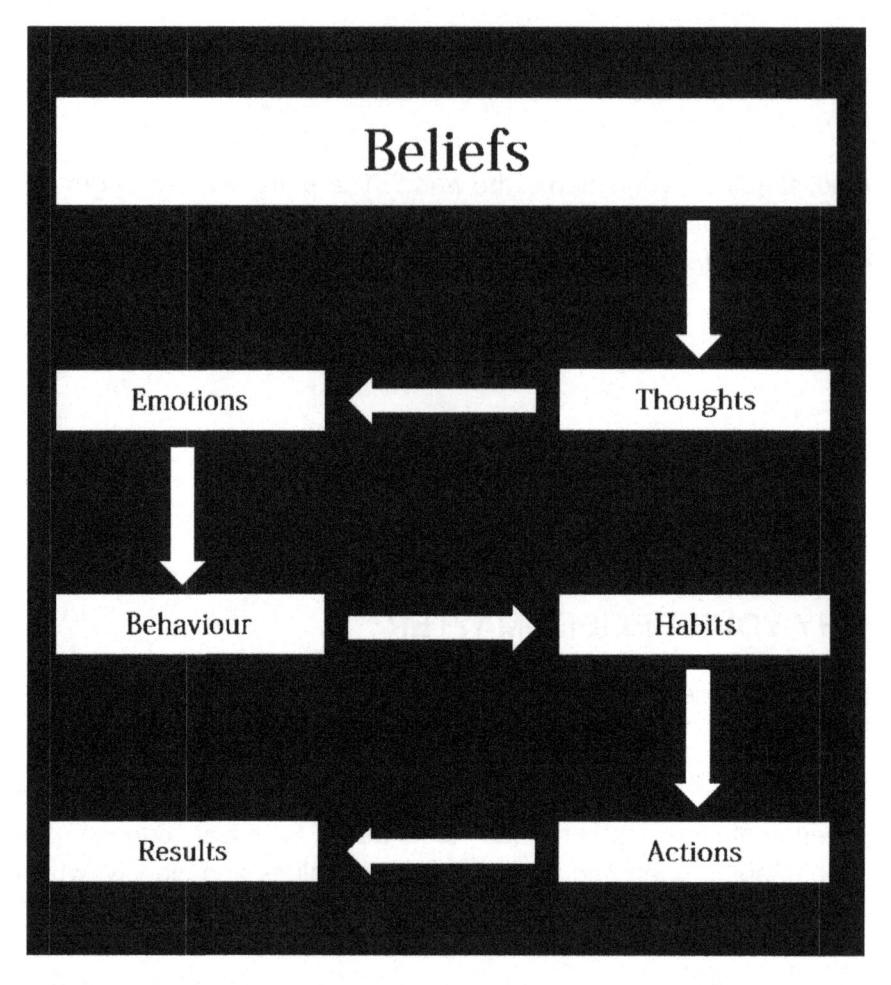

```
            Beliefs
               │
               ▼
Emotions  ◀──  Thoughts
    │
    ▼
Behaviour ──▶  Habits
                 │
                 ▼
Results   ◀──  Actions
```

Your conscious and subconscious beliefs affect your thoughts, which trigger emotions and feelings that influence your behaviour, which creates the habits that drive your actions leading to your results.

Why aren't you already healthy, wealthy and happy living the life of your dreams now? Your conscious and subconscious beliefs are holding you back. The world you have created is a result of your beliefs. It cannot be changed without changing your beliefs.

Even your best intentions, plans and knowledge cannot overcome doubt and uncertainty, which are all based on false beliefs.

The beliefs you choose for your life are more important than any goals because your belief determines the goals you will set, pursue and ultimately achieve.

If your beliefs are empowering enough, it will give rise to better goal setting and help you achieve those goals.

When you change your beliefs, you change what is possible.

Your beliefs form the blueprint for your life.

ARE YOUR BELIEFS TRUE?

They are for you but not necessarily for others. They may feel real because your emotions and feelings are real, but they're not necessarily true.

You have not consciously chosen most of your current beliefs, so how do you know they are true? What evidence do you have to support any belief?

Where did you get the information? Did you read about it or experience it? Is it based on other people's beliefs and opinions or the fundamental laws of the universe?

Your subconscious beliefs drive 90 per cent of your daily life, which directly impact every area of your:

- Judgement
- Values
- Attitude
- Decisions
- Behaviour
- Integrity
- Thoughts
- Emotions

- Habits
- Actions
- Health
- Wealth
- Results
- Lifestyle

All these elements affect the results you are getting – the good, the bad and the ugly. Ultimately your beliefs create your identity and your life.

If you want a different life with a different story, you need different beliefs.

'We are what we repeatedly do.'

Aristotle

When you believe something to be true, you rarely question or think about the validity of that belief. On one level, beliefs are your brain's way of making sense of and navigating a complex world.

Every individual has a different window into a reality filtered by their beliefs. Some beliefs are necessary for your survival, especially in the early years. *(I believe I might die if I walk off a cliff.)*

Other beliefs have been outgrown and no longer serve you, and can cause no end of pain, isolation and confusion. *(Don't talk to strangers.)*

You continue to live by your limiting beliefs even if they are detrimental to your success, lifestyle and well-being. Your brain continually seeks out people, events and circumstances that support your current beliefs. Psychology research over the years has shown that your mind is incredibly prone to error and bias.

Your brain wants safety and energy conservation first and foremost. Beliefs provide you with a level of certainty. Questioning and changing a belief poses a perceived threat to our psychological safety.

Beliefs are self-fulfilling prophecies and can also be addictive. Instead of facing the fear of change, you hold on to certainty even if the belief causes you physical or emotional discomfort.

BELIEF IS ONE THING; THINKING IS ANOTHER.

You may be manifesting what you subconsciously believe, not necessarily what you want. What you desire also has to match what you believe you deserve and are ready to receive. What you believe is what you will receive.

If you think, on a conscious level, of a successful outcome but believe, on a subconscious level, you are going to fail, your belief of failure will win!

If you want a different life with a different story, you need to make different choices.

LIMITING BELIEFS

Your false beliefs are the only obstacles that stand between your current position and your goals and dreams.

Limiting beliefs are the restrictor, the roadblock that causes you to operate at a lower level in most, if not all, areas of your life. What you are prepared to try is linked to your beliefs about your abilities around that issue.

If you don't change your limiting beliefs at both the conscious and subconscious levels, no amount of work, willpower or determination will change your life.

You will always default back to your underlying beliefs held to be true in your subconscious mind.

Your brain filters out anything that doesn't comply with your bias or the way you see life through your belief filters. Possibilities or impossibilities are based on your current beliefs – robbing you of opportunities you simply don't see, even if they are right under your nose.

Trying to change your life without changing your beliefs is like taking a shower in a raincoat – frustrating and uncomfortable. You have to change your false and limiting beliefs to change your life.

Your beliefs are one of the most potent forces on earth. Use their power to close the gap between where you are today and the future you are seeking.

The false belief of 'not being good enough' must have killed more dreams than anything else.

COMMON LIMITING BELIEFS (AKA EXCUSEITIS)

This shortlist of limiting beliefs affects most people to some degree in some areas of their lives. Feel free to add your own.

- I am too old.
- I am too young.
- Better safe than sorry.
- I don't have enough time.
- Money is hard to make.
- I can't do that.
- I am not enough.
- I am not smart.
- I don't have enough experience.
- Losing weight is a losing battle.

YOUR BELIEFS AND SUCCESS

- I can't make things happen.
- I am not talented.
- I will never find love.
- It's impossible to make money doing what you love.
- Earning money requires working hard.
- Money doesn't grow on trees.
- You just can't trust others with money.
- I will never be rich.
- Rich people are bad people.
- Money turns people rotten.
- You can't trust someone who has a lot of money.
- Money is not important to me.

Excuseitis are all the limiting excuses you have accepted as truth. If you look with intent, you will find someone, somewhere, who chose not to be limited by these beliefs or outside circumstances. If they can, you can.

A limiting belief may also be based on facts like you lack the skills needed to achieve your desired result. They are easy to acknowledge, identify and change. You can either learn the skills you need or employ someone who already has them.

What is your mind saying? *That's okay for you, but you don't understand how hard it is for me.*

☺

So there is your first limiting belief.

LIMITING MONEY BELIEFS

Example

Like a lot of people, I struggled with my beliefs about money. The topic of money was something I avoided because I wasn't comfortable talking about it.

Yet I still had a strong, overpowering desire to be wealthy, which caused me no end of pain and internal conflict for many decades.

My core belief was that money is limited and hard to make. I continued to attach supporting beliefs, such as, people argue over money, there is never enough money, money won't buy you happiness, there is more to life than money, and rich people are dishonest and selfish.

I associated emotional pain with money. I would make great money then get rid of it to fit back in with my beliefs and identity. I did this numerous times and couldn't work out why.

I knew this repeated behaviour had to stop, and to do that, I had to find out why I continued to self-sabotage. My work ethic wasn't the issue; I enjoyed being able to contribute.

Was it my choice of occupation, where I lived, the economy, the people I associated with? They may play a small part in the scheme of things, but the reality is, it was my false beliefs around money.

My brain created this intellectual, rational, even convincing self-justification of why I shouldn't be wealthy or why I was not successful at that moment.

Over time I developed a scarcity mindset to protect my core beliefs and justify my financial position.

> *However, it was based on false beliefs and flawed logic.*

ALTERNATIVE MONEY BELIEFS

Wealth and prosperity apply to all areas of your life: relationships, the work you do, your health, and money. But for now, let's focus on money. Money gives you the ability to fully experience life and help others.

If I say, 'I'm dedicated to having as much money as possible!' How would you judge me? You might feel uncomfortable being around me. You might think I am greedy.

But money is not the enemy; it is neutral. It is the beliefs and emotions you attach to it that cause you pain or pleasure.

> **Example**
>
> *Imagine a world without money. What would you exchange at the supermarket for your groceries or fuel at the local servo?*
>
> *You need to go to the doctor, but the doctor in your area will only exchange her services for someone who can build her a set of front stairs. Okay, a neighbour is a builder, so off you go to see him, and he will help if you can find him some new tires for his truck. You call the tire guy. He wants ... you get the picture.*

You can see the challenges of having to operate without legal tender. Money allows you to buy your groceries and clothes, take holidays, take care of your family and friends. Money provides options.

Start by being grateful for the role money plays in making your life easier and the opportunities it provides. Money is not the problem.

The issue is your false beliefs, combined with a lack of knowledge about earning, saving, investing and protecting your money.

Money won't solve all your problems, and it can create new problems of its own, but on balance, it's safe to say that money is a powerful problem-solving resource.

Money is a means of exchange. It is energy, and how much you attract is directly proportionate to how your energy (goods and services) positively impacts and helps others.

You receive money by filling a need, providing a service and bringing value to the marketplace. The marketplace determines the value people place on your products or service. As people's needs change, so does what they value and how much they are willing to pay for something.

Money enables you to give back to your community, to pick the charities and causes you believe in and want to support.

There is no shortage of money, and what you want is only a microscopic fraction of what's available. There is unlimited financial abundance available to anyone prepared to put in the mental effort to make it happen.

If you have emotional challenges – unresolved childhood traumas, issues with family, or difficulty forming and sustaining healthy relationships – money is not going to magically solve those problems for you. You still have to do the healing work required to deal with your emotional baggage to live a happier life.

CORE BELIEFS

Your core beliefs are your brain's operating software system. They provide a fixed set of pathways that automatically produce your daily thoughts and actions.

They are your North Star or compass point of reference for all conscious and subconscious decision-making.

Your core beliefs are surrounded and protected by layers of supporting beliefs. To change any belief, you must identify and remove the outer layers to reveal the core or central belief, like peeling an onion.

If you only work on the outer belief layers, your subconscious will still operate from the core belief, and it will be impossible to sustain permanent change in your thoughts, feelings, habits and actions.

SUPPORTING BELIEFS

You must filter through all the beliefs around a subject until you get a gut feeling for what those beliefs are and then what is at their core or heart.

Your list might be similar or different, but it must be *your* list. Next, spend time going through all your beliefs about *one* issue and keep narrowing it down until you get to the core belief that best fits your limiting belief.

There are no right or wrong core beliefs, as everyone has had different environments, backgrounds, teachers and parents. You also interpret the same event differently, so trust your instincts to go with what feels right.

Know what supporting beliefs protect and hold your core belief in place.

☺

Be wary of the beliefs and ideas you inherit.
They set false limits around your creativity and possibilities.

IDENTIFY YOUR LIMITING CORE BELIEFS

You were born with no sense of what you could or could not do. These beliefs were developed over time through your experiences. Now you need to identify and replace any limiting beliefs you have about your abilities.

Changing any belief starts first with an awareness of the limiting beliefs that are holding you back. Investigate any belief that causes suffering.

First, forgive yourself for adopting false beliefs, and permit yourself to go after your heartfelt desires, goals and dreams.

To find your limiting beliefs, make a statement about an area or something in your life:

- I would love to be fit but …
- I would love to find happiness but …
- I would love to find true love but …
- I would love to be wealthy but …
- I would love to travel the world but …
- I would love to start my own business but …
- I would love to …………… but ….

☺

Whatever comes up after 'but' is your limiting belief.

Recognise excuseitis as false beliefs. Don't allow your false beliefs to be an excuse for not achieving your dreams and goals.

If someone else has reached a similar result, they had to learn and grow to achieve their objective. So can you.

SUMMARY

- Every master was once a disaster.
- Change your beliefs, change your life.
- Success and failure are the results of your beliefs.
- Empowering beliefs light the pathway to success.
- It doesn't matter where you start; what's important is where you want to go.

ACTIONS

1. Accept that you are operating on false beliefs that you have unconsciously accepted as true. To start, pick one area of your life that you want to change that will have the biggest positive impact on your life. It could be a relationship, finances, health, career or self-development.
2. Briefly, without overthinking it, list 5 to 7 limiting beliefs that are stopping you from achieving your desired results.
3. Now write the opposite empowering beliefs.
4. Next, look for multiple examples where other people have achieved success similar to what you want.
5. You know that it's possible for others, so it's possible for you. You can learn to do anything. Study their methods and add your unique ADHD talents and 'different' approach to help you achieve your desired results.

Every master was once a disaster.
Break free from the cage of limiting beliefs.

ADHD ADDults

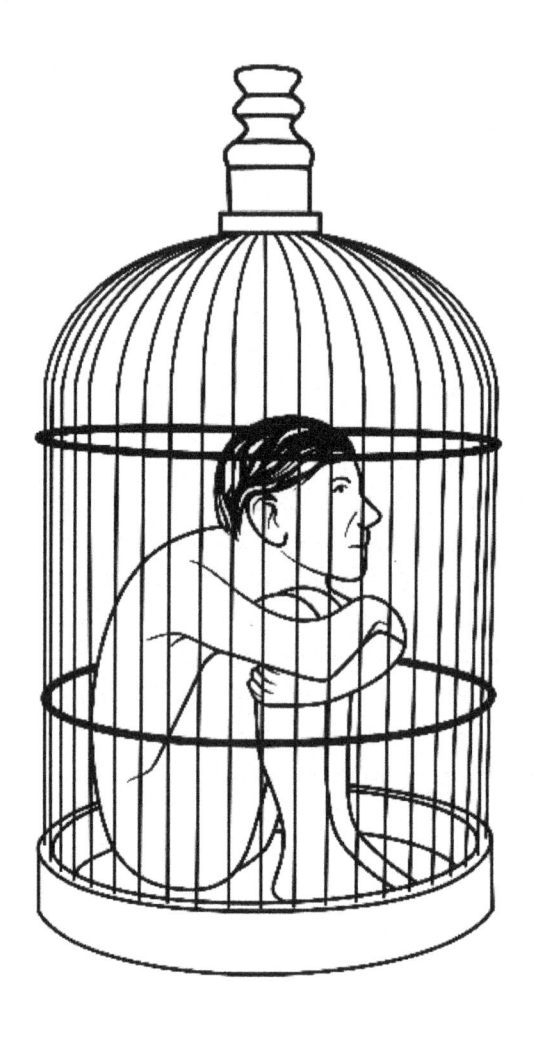

NOTES

5

WHY CHANGE YOUR BELIEFS?

Both belief and fear are something you hold in your mind as true with or without proof. Which one will you choose?

YOUR IDENTITY

You can't change your beliefs or life without altering your current identity. Your identity plays a critical role in the results you get in life.

Your current identity is the story you have repeatedly told yourself, which is based entirely on your old beliefs and the meaning you have given to the experiences throughout your life.

The entry point to shaping your identity lies in shifting your beliefs about yourself and about what is and isn't possible. For example, if you believe that you're not able to change your identity (i.e. a fixed belief system), then lasting change will not be possible, no matter how strong your desire is.

Why are you limiting yourself?

The tighter you cling to your old identity, the harder it is to build a new one. Your identity needs to be flexible like water, flowing around changing circumstances.

You have all the abilities within you to accomplish anything you desire. What fears are stopping you from claiming the life of your dreams?

Every fear and excuse you have can be traced back to your beliefs. Your brain will try to use fear and procrastination to stop you from changing your beliefs and life ... tell it to take a hike.

You have to recreate your reality and identity the way you want it to be. Choose your new identity, then start developing the beliefs, character traits, skills and values necessary to build that identity; link your new identity to your values and the primary goals you want to achieve.

RELEASE YOUR OLD IDENTITY

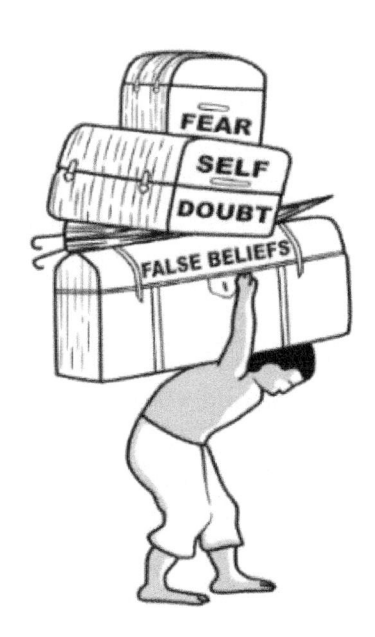

Dump the baggage, mate.

Living in alignment with your new beliefs helps you to get rid of the old excess baggage you are carrying around.

First, accept that, for some reason, you have developed this old identity, and now you want to create a new empowering one.

Without judgement, feeling guilty, blaming yourself or others, acknowledge that your identity was simply false beliefs and repeated patterns you developed without being aware that they were stopping you from achieving your dreams and goals.

Control your emotions and let go of any negative feelings, so you can focus your positive energy on your new identity, which will help you to achieve what you want.

To create your new identity, you have to be willing to let go of the old one.

If you are struggling to replace your old identity with its limiting behaviours, patterns and habits, ask these questions to help you get back on track.

- How would my new identity deal with this?
- What does my new identity look like?
- What mindset does my new identity have?
- What would my new identity do in this situation?
- How would my new identity turn this around?
- What actions would my new identity take?

SELF-BELIEF

Self-belief is the idea that you can figure things out and adapt to new situations. You can learn, you can grow, if you are placed in an unfamiliar situation you can work out how to navigate it, you can adapt and thrive, and you can handle whatever surprises life throws at you.

Your self-beliefs directly impact three interrelated areas:

- Self-worth
- Self-esteem
- Self-confidence

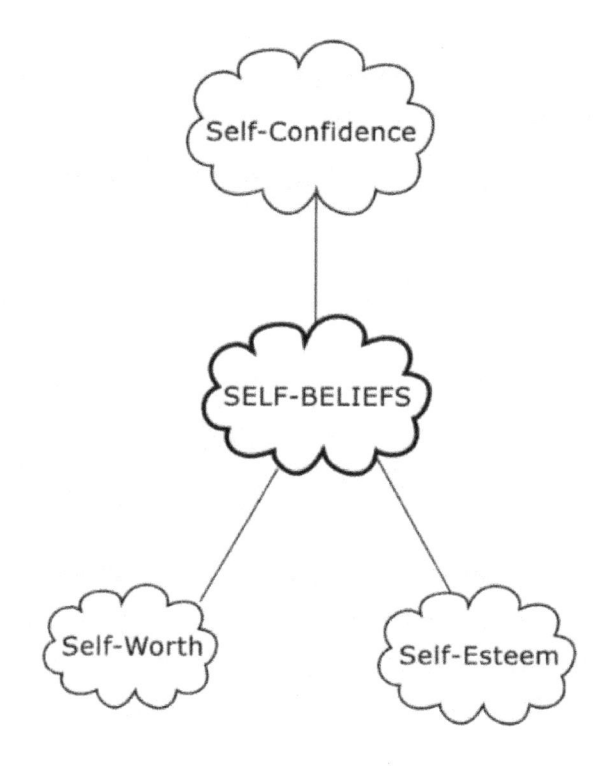

Self-belief is vital for your success.

SELF-WORTH

Your self-worth is a function of how you value yourself, your inner self, the value you place on your existence. Do you feel worthy of having a great, exciting and fulfilling life?

Example

Looking back, my first awareness of my self-worth came when I was about twelve years old and sent to a boarding school. I was dropped off one Sunday afternoon, and as I watched in amazement, my parent drove off.

My interpretation of this event was that there must be something wrong with me; my parents didn't want me in their life. I was unlovable. I was not worth the effort. While that may not have been true, these thoughts felt real to me at the time, and that is the belief I built my self-worth around.

My lack of self-worth directly affected my motivation; I couldn't see the point in striving for anything because I felt useless and unworthy, which affected my mental health. I only did as much as I had to do to survive.

My self-worth beliefs mixed with my false money beliefs made up a toxic cocktail of limiting beliefs.

- *I am not worthy of financial success.*
- *I can't support myself, let alone a family.*
- *I am not capable of achieving financial independence.*
- *I don't deserve to have a lot of money.*
- *I am not smart enough to become rich.*
- *I am not good enough.*

I was hell-bent on destroying my life, and I was very successful at doing just that.

To build self-worth you must first determine your highest core values and then create your definition of success.

SELF-ESTEEM

High self-esteem is thinking well of yourself, respecting yourself and your abilities and achievements in the outside world.

Low self-esteem makes it difficult to handle uncertainty, fear, stress and anger, leading to emotional extremes. You are also less likely to ask for help.

Self-esteem affects the decision-making process, which is already a challenge for your ADHD brain. It impacts your relationships and your overall well-being. You need high self-esteem to feel inspired to take on new challenges.

Self-esteem is the idea that you have worth and value. I am a worthy person; I deserve to be here. I have intrinsic value simply because of who I am.

SELF-CONFIDENCE

Self-confidence is the idea that you can accomplish things you want to achieve. I can choose to do that, I can talk to that person, I can write a book, I can do what I set my mind to.

Your environment, peer pressure, teachers and parents can have a massive impact on your current self-beliefs; statements like, what's wrong with you? Why did you do that, you idiot? Can't you do anything right? God, you're useless. You don't deserve ...

It is your interpretations about your value, skills, knowledge and abilities that determine the outcomes you expect.

But this reality isn't fixed. It is an image, a perspective you have in your mind.

Your conscious and subconscious self-beliefs directly impact three critical interconnected areas.

WHY CHANGE YOUR BELIEFS?

Self-belief is an internal game and totally under your control. As they say, it's all in your head. And it is.

Self-confidence is not an overall evaluation of yourself but a feeling of confidence and competence in specific areas, like sports, business or being a great partner or parent.

Don't link your self-confidence to your career, possessions, achievements, how you look or what other people think of you. This is a solo activity.

Self-confidence starts with keeping the promises you make to yourself. Don't underestimate the importance of honouring self-promises.

When you say you will get up at 5.30 a.m. to go do some exercise or study or do your morning rituals and don't do it, that unconsciously starts to undermine your beliefs about yourself.

Start with ten to fifteen minutes of physical activity, every day for thirty days. Or fifteen minutes of solo thinking time to go over your goals. Maybe only eating nineteen of the twenty doughnuts ... *only kidding, show some discipline and only eat eighteen, ha-ha!*

☺

Self-beliefs, not 'selfie' beliefs.

SELF-DOUBT

Before you can develop unwavering self-belief, you need to overcome self-doubt. Self-doubt hinders one's ability to take action and leads to massive procrastination and indecision. Your self-doubt is a limiting belief. It arises due to a perceived lack of confidence in your ability due to past failure or false beliefs.

Not believing in yourself allows doubt to creep into your life, which can start a flow of automatic negative thoughts (ANTs) that will undermine your self-belief. That will make it impossible for you to be fully committed to a task or goal and perform to the best of your ability.

Limiting self-beliefs about your self-worth and your self-image will prevent you from earning more than what you are conditioned and expect to earn at a subconscious level. Your ability to get what you want in your life will be compromised.

To overcome self-doubt, build your self-belief by recalling past events when you successfully handled challenges. This will help you to let go of self-doubt and enable the development of self-belief.

Even if you feel some doubt in the back of your mind, ignore it and proceed with taking action. When you take action despite uncertainty, your confidence will improve.

Just thinking positively and believing in yourself will not change anything. To support and strengthen your empowering beliefs it is essential to take consistent action.

It doesn't matter if you only take small steps to move towards your goals. As you advance and see minor improvements, you will feel motivated to take bigger steps towards your dreams.

Your identity, your self-belief, your self-confidence and your self-worth are based on your current core beliefs. To change a belief, you have to alter the false identity you acquired, moving closer to who you authentically are. Create a revised identity and story in line with your dreams and goals.

Knowing you are being guided and supported by a higher power, whatever you perceive that to be, greater than yourself, allows you to venture into uncertainty and push through the challenges.

Harness the power and influence of your self-belief. You will feel driven to act, delay gratification, and sustain it over longer periods.

Learn to see mistakes or setbacks as a part of the process and keep on going.

You must develop certainty in your new beliefs and confidence in your abilities. It must be a certainty derived from intelligent, conscious awareness, application and perseverance.

Positive self-belief is that feeling you have inside that you are capable of anything; you feel strong, confident and energised in the face of daily challenges and problems.

When you reach this stage of certainty, nothing can stop you. How long that takes will depend on the strength of your commitment, mental energy and how much consistent action you take.

True self-belief comes from developing the vision of whatever it is you need to believe you can do or be. You can teach yourself how to be confident, have self-belief, and behave in ways that maximise your chance of success.

An important part of self-belief comes from knowing your ADHD challenges and traits and being relaxed about them. When you accept them as part of you, you start to have more confidence in knowing that everyone has their own sh*t to deal with, and it is okay.

Self-belief stimulates reasoning, memory and creativity, making it possible to find good solutions.

SELF-SABOTAGE

Self-sabotage is self-inflicted destructive behaviour that erodes your self-confidence, self-esteem and self-worth. It prevents you from settings and achieving the goals you truly desire.

At first, you may not even notice that you're doing it.

You may procrastinate, repeatedly putting off critical issues you know you need to resolve. Every time you fail to complete something, it lowers your self-belief.

You consistently undermine your own efforts; you stop doing what you know needs to be done for no apparent reason. You are unable to move forward.

Maybe you start projects but never finish them. You let your important personal and career dreams die and never understand why.

Self-sabotage is often driven by negative thoughts and self-talk, where you tell yourself that you're not worthy of success, which fuels your self-sabotaging behaviours.

Without changing this behaviour, it can become a form of mental self-harm – invisible to the outside world but a constant torment and highly damaging to the individual.

There can be many different causes, but the effects are the same. You find yourself falling short of the goals you've set for yourself. Subconsciously you limit your potential for success.

Over time the failures build up and you question every decision, which further undermines your self-confidence.

STOP SELF-SABOTAGE

It starts will awareness. To stop self-sabotaging your life you need to be aware of the patterns of behaviour you have adopted.

Then look at the thoughts and the false beliefs behind your destructive behaviour. Question their validity; are they real or imaginary? Are they true in all cases?

Challenge your emotions by taking a detached view of the situation. Feel the emotion, but don't be controlled by it.

Identify the negative thoughts and replace them with positive, empowering thoughts.

To permanently defeat self-sabotaging behaviour you have to change your false, limiting beliefs to new empowering beliefs that align with your deepest dreams and goals.

SUMMARY

- Self-belief is vital for your success.
- Self-belief helps you relax and think clearly.
- Self-belief starts with honouring self-promises.
- Every fear and excuse you have can be traced back to your false self-beliefs.
- Your conscious and subconscious self-beliefs directly impact your self-esteem, self-worth and self-confidence.

ACTIONS

1. First, you need to design your new identity to become the person you need to be, achieve your goals and dreams, and fulfil your purpose.
2. Next, start developing and embedding new empowering beliefs, character traits, skills and values necessary to build that identity.
3. Identify what key things you would need to put in place and make happen right now, and what could you do physically as soon as possible to kick-start the process?
4. Build your self-belief by keeping the promises you make to yourself. Only make promises aligned with *your* values, major goals and life's purpose that you are committed to keeping.
5. Build your self-esteem and self-confidence by developing an empowering and supportive relationship with yourself. Start taking action, learning new skills and getting into the game.
6. Daily practice self-care over self-indulgence and reinforce your positive self-beliefs. It will provide you with endless energy, and you will feel like you are flowing with the river, not against it.

NOTES

6

CHANGING YOUR BELIEFS

Don't waste years of your life trying to change until you get your beliefs aligned with your goals and dreams.

BELIEF CHANGING

- **Awareness**. Constantly be aware of the beliefs behind the thoughts and feelings you experience.
- **Understanding**. Know those beliefs are not true or false until you give them meaning.
- **Detachment**. You are not your beliefs. See your beliefs from a calm, unemotional viewpoint.
- **Let go**. Release any beliefs and thoughts that don't support your goals and dreams.
- **Imprinting**. Find examples of successful people in your field. Study and model those people.
- **Strategies**. Develop and implement only those strategies that you judge to be right for you and discard the rest.

Because your conscious mind can only hold one thought at a time, either positive or negative, always choose the positive option.

Therefore the fastest and simplest way to change a belief is to hyper-focus your mental energy on installing new empowering beliefs that align with who you want to be and what you want to have and do.

Just ask, 'Do my current beliefs help me to achieve the results I want in my life?' If the answer is no, great. Invest all your energy in choosing and imprinting new positive beliefs that will support you.

Give your brain a reason to work with you by drip-feeding it dopamine along the way. Make the process of changing your beliefs an exciting and enjoyable adventure that is leading you towards amazing life experiences.

☺

Okay, first, just relax and change your beliefs about changing beliefs.

It is important to put in the effort to select and implement your new beliefs. Redesigning your empowering belief system and building a new sense of identity take time.

However, this will pay the biggest return on investment in your personal development journey by far, opening the door to unlimited possibilities.

Changing your beliefs happens at a subconscious level through deliberate conscious thoughts and actions.

Over time, with consistent action, your new belief displaces the old false belief. You are reprograming your brain. It is like installing a new program on a computer that you must learn to use effectively.

If you are struggling with really believing something, don't try and fool yourself. You know you don't have the ability ... yet.

Acknowledge the fact and believe you can learn, change, and develop the attitude and skills to achieve your goals and dreams. Build your new beliefs in smaller steps.

CHOOSE YOUR NEW BELIEFS

There is an infinite choice of beliefs, and you get to select which you want to have. No one else can do that for you. I'm just guiding you through the process.

Invest the time to select beliefs that align with and support your values, goals and dreams. Beliefs about money, health, career or business, relationships, your skills and abilities, and all the important areas in your life.

Ask what beliefs you need to have to achieve these outcomes. The vital thing is to have empowering beliefs supporting you instead of standing in your way.

EMPOWERING BELIEFS

The list of empowering beliefs is unlimited. This list is to get you thinking about what it is you want to do, be and have. Feel free to add your own.

- I am in perfect health.
- Mistakes are valuable.
- My best is yet to come.
- I have so much to offer.
- I can figure it out as I go.
- My success is inevitable.
- My destiny is in my hands.
- Money is a great resource.
- My wealth continues to grow.
- Learning is part of the process.

- I am the perfect age to succeed.
- If others have done it, I can do it.
- I have so much to be grateful for.
- The universe is 100% behind me.
- I can learn whatever I need to know.
- There is enough money for everyone.
- What I am are seeking is seeking me.
- I attract the right resources and people.
- I decide how I feel, no matter the situation.

INSTALLING NEW BELIEFS

Enjoy the challenge.

There is no one-size-fits-all method to installing new beliefs, but I can share what works for me. First, try what appeals to you, and then keep trying until you design the system that works best for you.

Let's start with the basics. Consistent repetition is the foundation of all progress. Whether it's a physical or mental activity you want to alter and improve, repetition is the glue that holds it together.

Develop an optimistic mindset, consciously supplying your mind with inspiring content. Read books that provide you with new perspectives and help you to take action.

Supercharge your mind with positive fuel throughout the day with inspiring books, videos, Ted Talks and podcasts.

Support your new beliefs with a constant flow of positive thoughts and prevent old beliefs from trying to take control.

> *Repetition is what makes champions and is a cornerstone of all successful people.*

AFFIRMATIONS

> *Affirmation without action is just a distraction.*

For many people, using affirmations to build positive beliefs is an effective way to start changing their beliefs. An affirmation is simply a short statement that you repeat silently or aloud if appropriate.

You don't have to believe them. It doesn't make any difference. Just keep repeating them, and they will imprint on the subconscious over time.

At first, you may doubt the truth of an affirmation because you know you currently lack the knowledge and skills needed to achieve your desired result. You don't have to force yourself to consciously believe the affirmation. Just relax, enjoy the process and trust your subconscious.

Keep your affirmations short. The shorter, the better, and the more impactful and quick to write or say, which is great for ADHDers. Your brain is smart and fully understands what these short statements are about.

There is no definite correct number of words. Try somewhere between two and seven. If you need more words, consider breaking it up into two declarations to get more clarity.

Always say your affirmation in the positive present tense, don't say you want to lose weight – instead, say something like – I am healthy. I am a runner or I am fitter.

This is not lying to yourself; it is an awareness that everything is produced in the mind first before it shows up in the physical world.

Then visualise it as already happening, run your mental video and experience the feelings of success, joy, excitement, gratitude or any positive feelings while saying your affirmation.

Your job is to be self-disciplined and repeat your affirmations at least once a day. Twice or three times is better and will help speed up the process.

Last thing at night and first thing in the morning, the mind responds well to the new beliefs, visions and behaviours you want to experience.

To mould your subconscious mind requires conscious effort and repetition before it becomes your new default belief. Don't aim for perfection. Consistent progress is far more important and productive. Three steps forward, one step back.

Make it a ritual. Practice your affirmations and actions with feeling, and repeat this throughout the day as though you are learning a new skill or building a new muscle. This must be felt and experienced.

Remember, at first, you don't have to believe them; it doesn't make any difference. Just keep repeating them, and they will imprint on the subconscious over time. Just try it for ninety days.

It does not matter how often you say an affirmation; it will not make a difference in your life if you don't imagine it or feel it.

SUMMARY

- Different beliefs equal a different life.
- Affirmations must be backed with action.
- Your core beliefs are your brain's operating software system.
- Empowering beliefs are the 'supercharger' of your life.
- Align your new beliefs with your values, goals and life's purpose.

> *Knowledge brings awareness, but without reprograming your subconscious mind, your life can't change. New beliefs are required and acquired by doing real-life exercises; reading by itself will achieve zero.*

ACTIONS

There are numerous ways to change your beliefs. I have provided two options that have worked for me. Try them or seek out alternative methods.

OPTION 1

New empowering belief

I AM ALREADY THAT WHICH I WANT TO BE.

The belief behind this statement is that everything you need to achieve your goals and dreams already exists within you and in the universe.

All the support, every answer, or solution you need to change your life already exists in the superconscious mind, which you have access to through your subconscious mind during meditation and sleep.

You accept that your intellect can't solve all your problems and ask infinite intelligence to provide the solutions you seek and believe you will receive them. Then it is up to you to get to work, making them a reality in the physical world.

Remember, you have to trust in a wisdom and a power that transcends your understanding. Like the wind, you can't see it, but you can feel its effect.

OPTION 2

8 STEPS TO CHANGING YOUR BELIEFS

1. Select ONE limiting core belief that stands between you and your goals and dreams. Choose the belief that will have the biggest positive impact on your life. It could be your physical or mental health, career, or financial situation.
2. Choose ONE empowering core belief that will move you closer to your values, goals and dreams. You know which one will have the most impact on your overall life and well-being.
3. Write your new empowering belief as a positive, exciting affirmation combined with matching images of the new empowering belief. Give it total focus; get absorbed in, even obsessed with, it. Wrap your mind and spirit around it until you feel it becoming like a second skin.
4. Repetition is essential for reinforcing your new empowering belief until it becomes a reality. Use consistent repetition to program the new belief into your subconscious until it becomes your default belief. Repetition of the same affirmations leads to belief, and once that belief becomes a deep conviction, things begin to happen.
5. Accept the new belief. Focus on it. See yourself acting in alignment with your new belief and identity. Stop doing anything associated with your old belief. Stay neutral and stop reacting to your past belief. The belief is gone when there is no emotional attachment to the words you use to describe the old belief.
6. Be aware when you feel a strong negative emotion, catch yourself thinking a thought that is limiting, or find yourself in a repetitive, habitual loop that does not serve you. STOP and hit the DELETE button. Flood your mind with positive affirmations and images of your empowering belief.

CHANGING YOUR BELIEFS

7. Next, take massive action in areas you had avoided working on due to false fears caused by your limiting belief. Continually look for evidence that supports your new empowering belief.
8. Continuously listen to audiobooks and YouTube videos that support the new beliefs you are installing into your subconscious mind. This is vital in stopping your old thoughts and beliefs from trying to maintain control of your ADHD brain's pathways.

Example

My limiting core belief was 'I am not enough', supported by other limiting beliefs, 'I am not capable', 'I am not smart enough', 'I am not worthy'.

My new empowering belief was 'I AM ENOUGH'.

I write the following affirmations every morning to strengthen my 'I AM ENOUGH' belief.

I am kind; I am smart.
I am happy; I am healthy.
I am worthy; I am capable.
I am successful; I am wealthy.
I am generous; I am grateful.

I AM ENOUGH

Go to www.adhdadults.com/resources to download your bonus worksheets.

NOTES

7

YOUR BIG S.I.M.P.L.E. GOALS

> *'Write it so a six-year-old child can understand it …'*
>
> **Albert Einstein**

Curiosity, creativity and learning are essential to ADHDers, and without them you become depressed.

It is vital that you choose goals that allow you to lead an exciting, fulfilling and adventurous life while contributing your unique talents to the world.

Goals give your ADHD brain structure and clear objectives to achieve.

Always keep things as simple as possible. That allows you to focus all your energy on your major goals, making you more effective. Too many goals stress your brain, causing procrastination and feelings of overwhelm.

Don't overthink or overcomplicate your goals or the process. Complexity is the killer of goals. It's about enjoying the big and small dopamine rewards along the way.

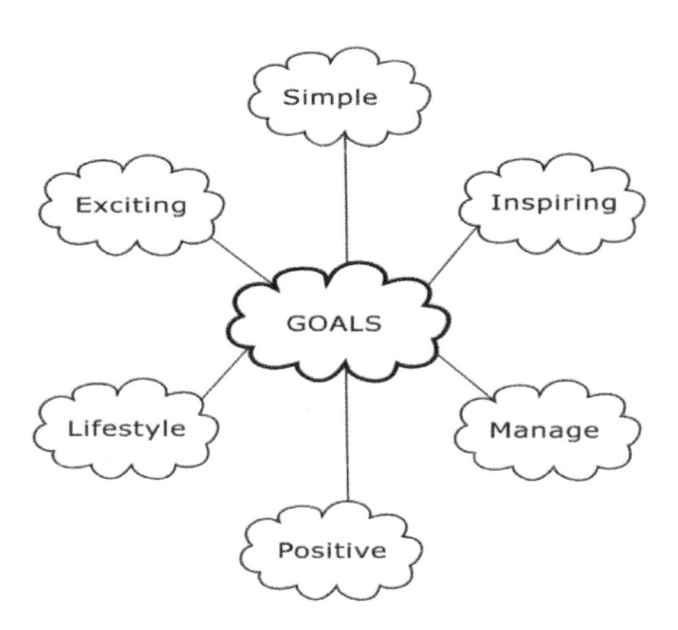

SIMPLE

Simplify your major goal. Break it down to its most basic components. You must describe it in a way that most people get it, quickly and easily. If you have to explain it in great detail, it's too complex.

Clearly describe the exact result you want to achieve and the timeline to achieve the goal. It must be black and white, with no grey areas you can use as an excuse. Either you reached your goal, or you didn't. Don't bullsh*t yourself.

INSPIRING

You have to be inspired by your goals. You need the motivation and drive from being inspired to achieve them. Design your compelling future. If you aren't truly inspired by your dreams, you will go looking for the next bright shiny object, or when the sh*t hits the fan, you will walk away and give yourself a perfectly valid excuse as to why it didn't happen. You must be inspired to inspire others.

MANAGE

Be the observer of how your life is going. Reward yourself regularly for sticking with the systems and process. Continually refine and manage your strategies, systems and timelines to help you achieve your goals. If something isn't working, change your approach, don't change your goal.

Use numbers to measure, discover, manage and modify. Like, going from a 38-inch waist to a 34-inch waist in ninety days, three twenty-minute exercise sessions a week, saving $1,000 for a holiday, meditating for ten minutes, a sixteen-hour fast.

ADHDers need deadlines or it won't get done. Set *starting* and *finishing* times for each goal. Be accountable and work to your time schedule. Add an extra 20 per cent to the time you think it will take, then try and complete the task or project under that time.

Monitor to see if you are showing up. Measure to see if you're spending time on the things that are important to you. Developing the beliefs, behaviours and habits needed to reach your goals is a vital step. Learn to love the process as much as the results.

POSITIVE

Start with a positive mindset. Give fear and doubt the day off. Suspend all your old beliefs.

Make sure your goals are a positive experience for everyone concerned. You live in an abundant universe. There is enough for everyone.

Positively state your goals. Reframe goals such as 'I want to stop eating junk food' into more a positive statement like 'I am eating healthy and nutritious food', or 'I want to stop the negative chatter in my head' into 'I am mentally stronger and learning to control my thoughts'.

LIFESTYLE

Set sustainable goals that will give you the things, experiences and lifestyle you want. There is no point in setting goals if they are not aligned with your core values or conflict with your desired lifestyle.

Either you won't achieve your goal, or if you do, it will be difficult to maintain long term, and it won't be fulfilling. Get your beliefs, values, goals and lifestyle aligned.

EXCITING

Life is meant to be an adventure; don't choose your goals to match what anyone else is doing. Of the seven billion-plus people on our planet, no two people share the same DNA. Why should you share identical goals?

Allow yourself to jump into areas that are an excellent match for your ADHD interests, desires and talents. Enjoy the process and the journey as much as your achievements.

YOUR GOAL-SETTING OPPORTUNITY

Make sure any major goal is worthy of your time and energy. A lot of people waste their most precious resources on insignificant goals.

You are the ultimate learning machine. From the day you were born, you have grown and evolved into the person you are today. In the early stages, you had little choice in what you learned or your path of development.

Sometimes the growth has been painful; sometimes, it has been enjoyable. Now you get to choose what you want to learn and what interests you want to develop to a higher level.

When setting your goals remember true fulfilment comes from your evolution, who you become. Goals and material things are just one part of the picture that adds to your overall happiness and fulfilment. When you reach any goal, it's not the end; it is who you become.

Embrace your ADHD individuality – live outside the cage others have built for you. People around you might say, 'Get a real job', or 'Just grow up'. 'Stop taking risks.' 'Stop enjoying all that stimulation.' 'Stop wanting to do your own thing.' 'You've gotta learn to conform, to play the game, to calm down and relax.'

Emergency medical personnel, firefighters, fighter pilots, police officers, engineers, inventors, artists and entrepreneurs thrive on not being held captive by other people's limitations. No matter what you do with your life, some people won't be happy about it; that's okay because it's your life, not theirs.

ADHD ADDults

Build your own exciting and compelling future that draws you forward to your goals and dreams.

5 LIFE ELEMENTS

In the interests of simplicity, I have provided the following five life elements to consider. I encourage you to think for yourself and add or delete as you see fit. No one can tell what is right for you; that is your job.

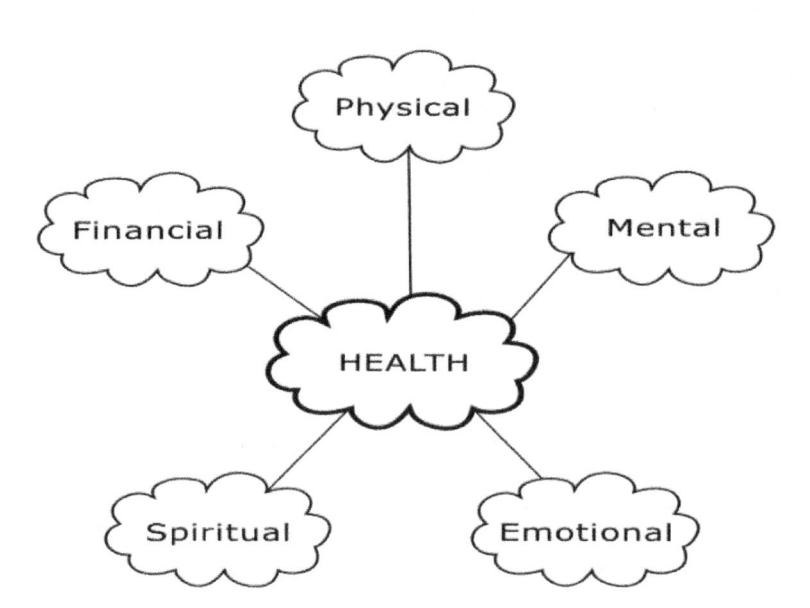

```
           Physical
Financial           Mental
           HEALTH
Spiritual           Emotional
```

YOUR BIG S.I.M.P.L.E. GOALS

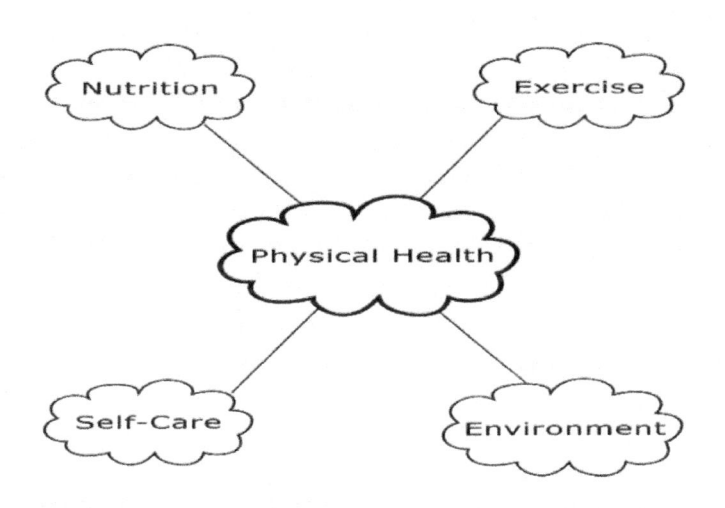

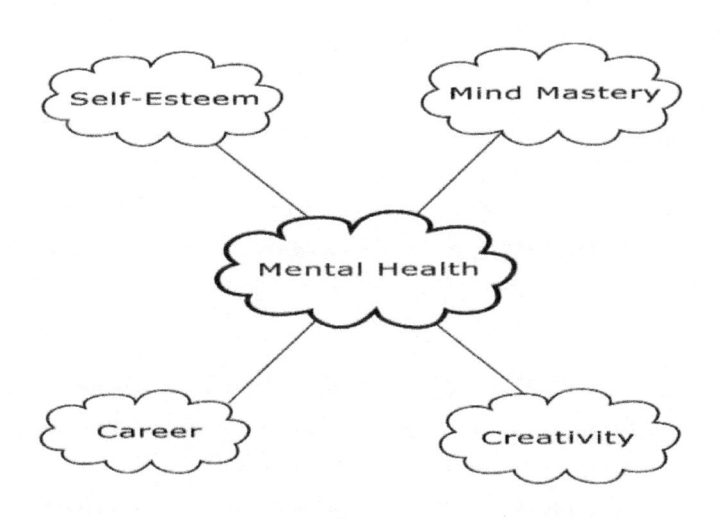

- Nutrition
- Exercise
- **Physical Health**
- Self-Care
- Environment

- Self-Esteem
- Mind Mastery
- **Mental Health**
- Career
- Creativity

ADHD ADDults

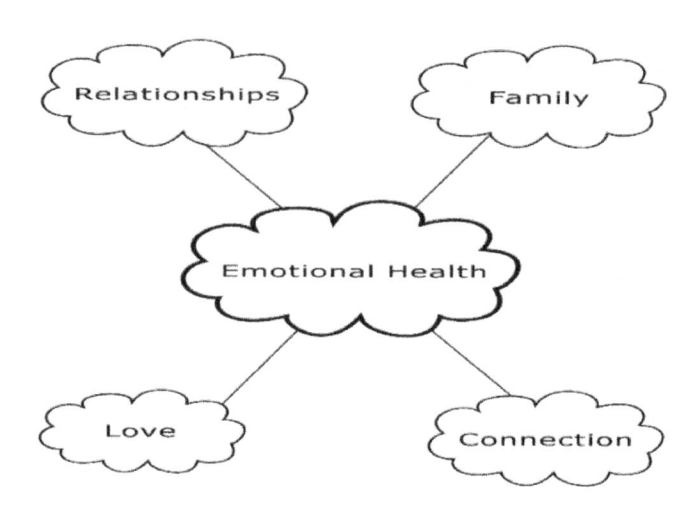

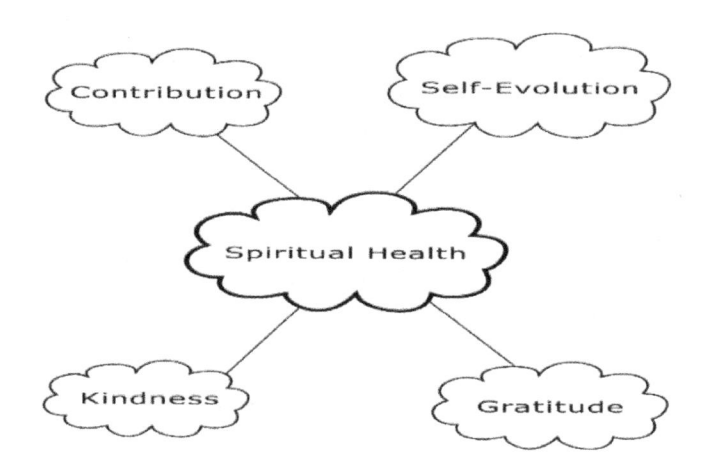

- Relationships
- Family
- Emotional Health
- Love
- Connection

- Contribution
- Self-Evolution
- Spiritual Health
- Kindness
- Gratitude

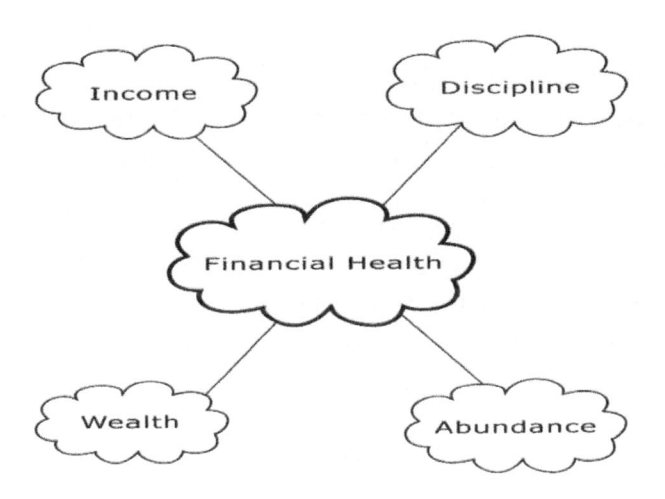

```
         Income              Discipline
             \              /
              Financial Health
             /              \
         Wealth              Abundance
```

Now apply your ADHD talents of super-focus and imagination to get the party started.

To avoid confusion and feeling overwhelmed, start with just one major goal from each of these elements that will make the most significant difference in your life in the next 30–365 days when you accomplish it.

Before you write your list of goals and dreams, you must suspend *all* your current beliefs. Nothing is off the table.

THE BASICS

Develop a vision of how you want your life to be, who you want to become, what you want to achieve, and what things and experiences you want to have.

Identify your needs so you can consciously select goals that meet these needs. By knowing and owning your needs, you will be more motivated to work out how to achieve them through goal setting.

Choose what you want to create, hold on to that image as clearly and as often as you can and avoid the shiny object syndrome (**SOS**) at all costs.

To help get clarity and discover your individual goals, ask yourself the following questions. The answers are your reasons behind your WHY.

1. Who do I want to become?
2. What do I want to acquire?
3. What do I want to accomplish?
4. What do I want to experience?

Example

I will use my physical health goals. I chose health and fitness to focus on first because I believe I need all the endurance, vitality and energy I can generate to achieve all my other major goals.

Who do I want to become?

- *I want to be self-disciplined and 100% responsible for my nutrition and lifestyle choices.*
- *To be aware and grateful for my mind and body's amazing abilities.*
- *Strong and healthy at any age.*
- *The best version of me.*

What do I want to acquire?
- *Gym membership that has a large range of equipment and is easy to get to.*
- *Buy some weights to have a home.*
- *Build a small home gym for convenience.*

> *What do I want to accomplish?*
> - *To have my body fat under 20%.*
> - ***Take exceptional care of my mind and body.***
> - ***Exercise every day for at least fifteen minutes.***
> - ***Intelligent nutrition.***
> - *Improved strength, endurance and flexibility.*
>
> *What do I want to experience?*
> - *Exceptional energy and vitality.*
> - *The positive benefits of self-discipline.*
> - *A long, healthy and active life.*
> - *Maximum brainpower and directed focus.*
> - *Intelligent and beneficial dopamine rewards.*
> - *I want to live in a healthy environment.*
>
> *I used these affirmations for my physical health goals.*
> - *I am exceptionally healthy.*
> - *I am the perfect age.*
> - *I am living with renewable energy and vitality.*
> - *I am focused yet relaxed.*
> - *I am enjoying my active lifestyle.*

ACHIEVING YOUR GOALS

> *Life is a huge university, and you can learn anything if your belief, desire and commitment are strong enough.*

For ADHDers, goal achievement needs to be structured to provide regular mini dopamine feel-good moments, so you can enjoy the journey by sticking to your systems and working through the processes each day on the way to your goals.

There will be a price to pay. You have to determine what that is. Long hours, 5 a.m. starts, isolation, relocation, delayed gratification, your goals, your list. Only you can decide if your goals and dreams are worth the price.

Now that you have set some goals, create a vision board or PowerPoint presentation of what you will achieve. Have clear visual pictures for your mind to work with. Write a clear description of the person you want to become.

Then, develop a structure with systems, daily routines, and habits. If you're a writer, make sure you write 365 words every day. If you want to get healthy, exercise for fifteen minutes minimum every day. If you want to acquire a new skill, invest thirty minutes learning from the best in that field.

Reverse engineer by starting from the final result you want. Work back from there and write down the steps needed to accomplish the goal as best you can. Each major goal may have many steps. It doesn't have to be perfect, as it will need adjustment when life gets in the way.

Break each of your major goals into smaller sub-goals with milestones that are easy to achieve and don't trigger feelings of overwhelm. Be okay with small successes to start with; this will build momentum and help you progress to bigger goals over time.

Overcome shiny object syndrome and stay focused on one thing until you achieve the results you want. Learn one thing effectively until you become a true master.

You also need to reward yourself along the way for each milestone you accomplish. This is a vital part of staying the course on longer-term goals. Without rewards, your ADHD brain starts to procrastinate and defaults back to **SOS.**

YOUR BIG S.I.M.P.L.E. GOALS

Keep a success journal and write up your successes each day, no matter how small. It will help you stay on course and build your self-confidence. You will feel more in control of your life. It will also help to keep you accountable.

You can start with something as simple as you exercising for fifteen minutes. You did the washing. You read for twenty minutes. The act of acknowledging your small successes will motivate you to up the ante on your major goals.

Every action affects your subconscious beliefs and, subsequently, your confidence. Keeping self-promises builds self-belief and self-confidence.

Doing something every day builds momentum and keeps the doubts away.

Just starting can get you motivated. Focus on how it will make you feel when it's completed, instead of the actual task. Identify the best time to work on your tasks and schedule blocks of time where you won't be distracted.

You will have setbacks. Keep going! You are on your way towards building positive beliefs, behaviours and habits that will lead to you achieving your goals and dreams. Learn to embrace the challenge; engage with it instead of avoiding it. It builds strength and confidence.

If it will take several years, you might want to create a series of projects or sub-goals that will take ninety days or less – any longer, and it's hard to stay motivated.

Aircraft are off course for over 90 per cent of their flight yet still arrive at their destination. Pilots and systems make constant course corrections to compensate for a multitude of issues that occur during the flight.

Achieving your goals is the same – to reach your destination you will have to adjust your course many times to compensate for getting blown off course by any unforeseen events. By all means, make adjustments in response to the conditions you encounter, but don't change your destination.

How you achieve your goals may change, but the destination, the mission, remains the same. Delays are not denials.

You need to feel that you are continually improving, even if it is only in small steps. They will compound over the weeks, months and years ahead.

To achieve your goals in life, regularly identify gaps in your knowledge and skills that could hold you back from achieving your goals. Then set educational sub-goals to fill in those gaps, and work step by step to achieve them. Whatever you need to know, someone else has already done it, so follow their blueprint, modify it to suit your specific goals, and learn from your own experiences.

Complexity is the enemy of action.
Keep it SIMPLE

SUMMARY

- Set S.I.M.P.L.E. goals.
- Make sure they are your goals.
- Remember, you can learn anything.
- Invest your time and energy where you get the highest ROL 'return on life'.
- When setting goals, avoid tying them to the performance or willingness of other people.

Value progress over perfection.

ACTIONS

Writing out clear goals with specific steps gives your brain structure and a road map to follow. Make them crystal clear ... black and white.

1. Go for what you truly want – Too many people make compromises with themselves. Do not do that. Go for *exactly* what you want and nothing less. Find a way, not an excuse.
2. Choose one major goal from each of the five elements that inspires you.
3. Create your whiteboard, vision board, or PowerPoint presentation.
4. Use the pleasure of achieving your goals and the fear of mediocrity and boredom to provide the fuel and the drive to keep you going when the sh*t hits the fan.
5. Work on one goal at a time, and prepare all the materials and information you need to work on your goal before beginning. Know what you want to achieve and set a timer.
6. List the skills and knowledge you need to reach each goal, and buy one book and study it to implement at least 5 key points to help you achieve the goal ... then repeat. Each time you read the same book you find ideas that you missed the first time.
7. Find the people and resources you need to achieve your goal ... ASK for help.
8. Develop your daily rituals, routines and habits. Write a one-page action plan and review it each morning and evening.
9. Practise JFT ... *just for today,* do whatever it takes.

10. Set challenging timelines, knowing it might take longer than expected.
11. Choose progress over perfection.
12. Start and never, never stop!

Go to www.adhdaddults.com/resources. for additional resources, worksheets and examples to help kick-start the process.

NOTES

8

YOUR THOUGHTS

'Change your thoughts and you change your world.'

Norman Vincent Peale

WHAT ARE YOUR THOUGHTS?

Your thoughts are potent and can alter your world and potentially the world as a whole. Everything created started as a thought in someone's mind – the good, the bad and the ugly.

They are mental perceptions – shaped by your life experiences and beliefs about yourself and the world around you.

Why are your thoughts so critically important?

Your thoughts have the power to work for you or against you. Your thoughts will make or break your world.

Your ADHD thoughts are longer, stronger and harder to control. Your brain becomes hardwired for repetition, and rumination sets in. When that happens, it's even harder to stop your cycling thoughts.

But it is possible.

You have this amazing gift of free thought, and by choosing better, positive thoughts, you can change your world. Your thoughts have the immense power to deliver your dreams and desires.

Your thoughts are energy, and like sparks from a fire, they can fade quickly. To give your positive thoughts staying power, you need to capture them and act on them quickly.

THOUGHTS ARE NOT FACTS

Don't believe every thought you have.

Where do your thoughts come from, and are they your own? Or are they drawn from an infinite universal warehouse of thought bubbles?

A bit like Amazon, where your brain goes shopping for thoughts that fit your beliefs, perceived environment, and expectations, they are delivered instantly, and they're free!

Universal law says you must become what you predominately think about. Your subconscious doesn't know or care if the thought is true or false. It merely accepts whatever you are thinking.

According to the National Science Foundation, an average person has about sixty thousand thoughts per day. Your ADHD brain may well exceed this.

Of those, 80 per cent are negative, and 95 per cent are repetitive thoughts. You think negatively more than you think positively. Cognitive-behavioural therapists have a term for it: automatic negative thoughts (ANTs).

ANTs

Automatic negative thoughts (ANTs) are random, negative thoughts you have. Your brain thinks predominantly negative thoughts for a good reason, it wants to keep you safe.

However, most automatic negative thoughts (ANTs) are false alarms that are disempowering, cloud your judgement and cause chronic stress, which impacts your brain.

Aaron Beck, MD, in the 1960s gave automatic negative thoughts the acronym of *ANTs*.

Daniel Amen, MD, is a psychiatrist and bestselling author. While he didn't coin the term ANTs, he certainly did raise its importance in his great bestselling book *Change Your Brain, Change Your Body*.

Below is his list of negative ANTs

1. **All or nothing** – It is black or white thinking; you think everything is good or all bad.
2. **Always thinking** – This is when you think in words that overgeneralise, such as *always, never, every time* or *everyone*.
3. **Focusing on the negative** – you only see the negative aspects of situations even when there are plenty of positives.
4. **Thinking with your feelings** – Thoughts like this occur when you have a feeling about something and you assume it is correct, so you never question it. Feelings can lie too.
5. **Guilt beating** – Thinking in words like *should, must, ought to*, and *have to* are typical with this type of ANT, which involves using excessive guilt to control behaviour.
6. **Labelling** – When you call yourself or someone else names or use negative terms to describe them, you have a labelling ANT in your brain.
7. **Fortune telling** – Predicting the worst even though you don't know what will happen is the hallmark of the fortune-telling ANT.

8. **Mind reading** – When you think that you know what somebody else is thinking even though they have not told you, and you have not asked them.
9. **Blame** – Of all the ANTs, this one is the worst. Blaming others for your problems and taking no responsibility for your own successes and failures is toxic thinking. It's believing you are a victim and that you are powerless to change your behaviour. Quit blaming others and take responsibility for your actions.

The negative effects of constant automatic negative thinking include:(13)

- Subconscious negative thought patterns
- Depletes beneficial brain chemicals like the feel-good neurotransmitters serotonin and dopamine
- Slows the production of brain-derived neurotrophic factor (BDNF), a protein required for new brain cell formation
- Shrinks the size of the brain but enlarges the amygdala, the brain's fear centre
- Increases the risk of psychiatric and neurodegenerative diseases
- Accelerates the brain's ageing process

Practise awareness of your thoughts by listening to your feelings. Are you feeling negative or positive?

- Use positive affirmations to replace the negative thoughts.
- Use your journal to track your negative thought patterns.
- Use positive affirmations to replace persistent negative thoughts.

Noticing your automatic negative thoughts and employing simple techniques to challenge and control them is worth the effort.

Turning off an unending flow of negative mental chatter is one of the best things you can do for your overall mental health.(14)

PETs

This is a technique I came up with to help me defeat my ANTs.

When I notice an ANT ... automatic negative thought floating around my head, I call up my PETs ... positive empowering thoughts. I find the opposite positive, empowering thought to the ANT I am experiencing to blow it away.

> *'A man is but the product of his thoughts. What he thinks, he becomes.'*
>
> **Mahatma Gandhi**

You can use several techniques to reduce the number of thoughts that your mind thinks per day; the best methods that provide a real solution and many benefits are exercise, meditation and focused concentration on a single task in an uncluttered and distraction-free space.

When the stream of thoughts slows down, you will be able to focus your mind on what you are doing without being distracted, and your mind can work better at studying, solving problems, making plans, doing your work and so on. The mind becomes a much more efficient and useful tool.

Learning to consistently and consciously change your thoughts is powerful enough to change your life.

AWARENESS

> *If you realised how powerful your thoughts are, you would never think another negative thought.*

Awareness of what you are constantly thinking is the key to gaining control over your mind and your life.

Your thoughts create your reality over time. There is a gap between when you think of something and when it starts manifesting in the physical world.

YOUR THOUGHTS AND SUCCESS

Ninety per cent of the time, your subconscious thoughts are the same each day, and that is why your life doesn't change.

Something more than hard work is necessary: namely, creative thinking and a firm belief in your ability to execute your ideas. All successful people have succeeded through their thinking.

Your thoughts produce your reality.

The immense power of your thoughts will lead to your decisions, habits and behaviour. This will ultimately lead to you achieving (or not achieving) your goals.

Call it storytelling, internal dialogue, self-talk or the unconscious dialogue in your head (whether you are aware of it or not). The things you say to yourself about yourself have a massive influence on your behaviour.

Up to now, your capacities have been constrained by constant inner struggles. The internal battle is between the voices in your head.

Your calm universal mind and your lunatic roommate. You know the one that says, you're stupid; you're useless; no, that will never work; you could never do that.

The same one that insults you at every opportunity. You are locked up with a maniac who can ruin anything without a moment's notice. This is one seriously disturbed alter ego that continually changes its mind, has conflicting views on most subjects, and is emotionally overreactive.

If you lived with someone like that, you would tell them to move out. Yet you allow this lunatic to live rent-free in your most valuable real estate, your mind. Think of how much time and energy is wasted on your unwanted roommate.

Most times, this voice is wrong. What's the cost associated with that in all the different areas of your life? This maniac thrives on fear and uncertainty, has an opinion on everything, knows nothing, and comes up will the wildest worst-case scenarios.

Why do you continue to ask for and take advice from this lunatic? Are you addicted to repetitive thinking, which releases chemicals to the brain like alcohol and drugs?

You only challenge the voice in your head when the fear of suffering under its faulty logic is greater than the fear of being without its illusion of protection.

You will defy the flawed logic when you realise it is based on fear. Your desire to get out of pain and be happy will propel you to personal freedom from the voice in your head.

Whether you realise it or not, the voice in your head has been doing the very best it could to guide you to be happy and prosperous. However, it has been operating on an outdated set of beliefs that no longer apply.

Its intent has always been for your safety and happiness. However, its methods have become exaggerated to the point of being abusive.

GOOD THINKING

The purpose of thinking is to understand your world as best you can. Your mind has evolved to think so that you can better adapt to your environment and make smarter decisions on how to survive, live and thrive.

Thinking plays a vital role in solving the personal problems you experience in your own life. Everything from relationships to work requires some element of thinking and problem-solving.

Thinking is the only way to sort facts from fiction, truth from lies. Undoubtedly, it is the greatest challenge facing us as individuals living in this modern information and misinformation age.

No skill is more valuable and harder to come by than the ability to think through problems. Poor initial decisions are one of the reasons you're so busy.

With flawed thinking, a large chunk of your time is spent correcting mistakes. On the other hand, good thinking produces better initial decisions and frees up time and energy.

However, while thinking does come with many benefits to your survival and evolution, it can also be two-sided.

OVERTHINKING

☺

Overthinking is the art of creating solutions to problems that don't exist.

Many with ADHD or other mental challenges like depression, anxiety disorder, or OCD are excessive thinkers. You may dwell on problems to unhealthy levels, especially about past events or things you have little control over.

You must learn to control and limit your thinking.

Overthinking is usually misdirected energy. You can waste a lot of time and energy going over things. Learn to identify when your thinking is serving your interests and needs and when it is leading you down the rabbit hole.

If you can make this distinction, you have already won half the battle with your thoughts.

Controlled thinking is your most important survival tool; it allows you to adapt to changing environments. Your ability to survive and thrive depends on figuring things out and making sense of the world.

DIFFERENT THINKING

'The world you have created is a product of your thinking; it cannot be changed without changing your thinking ...'

Albert Einstein

Changing your life requires different thinking.

Too often, you drift towards a predetermined response laid out for you by society. Society says if you're in this situation, do this. Different thinking allows you to choose what is truly best for you.

Your ADHD brain allows you to approach problems from different angles. Take in facts, statistics and information, analyse and question the reasoning behind them, and adapt them to your particular situation or challenge.

The barrier to different thinking is confirmation bias – your brain doesn't want change and will look for opinions, knowledge and views that confirm your worldview or belief is false.

The power of different thinking is the essence of creativity. By learning to think differently, you will find that your creative skills improve. This leads to powerful problem-solving abilities.

Different thinking will change how you feel and view the world. As you understand and implement this concept, you will start to go beyond your previous limitations.

CALM THINKING

> *'Thinking is nothing but the process of asking and answering questions.'*
>
> **Tony Robbins**

Imagine what would happen if you were free to focus only on the events currently taking place. You would have no noise going on inside. If you lived like this, you could do anything.

Your capabilities would be exponentially greater compared to anything you've ever experienced. If you could bring this depth of awareness and clarity to everything you do, your life would have to change.

Calm thinking involves letting go of what you want to believe and evaluating and embracing current reality.

When you do your research and finally lay out what you believe to be the facts, you will probably be surprised by what you uncover. It might not be what you were expecting, but chances are it is closer to the truth.

CAPTURE YOUR THOUGHTS

Cognitive scientists believe that working memory is one of the major components of intelligence. Working memory is like the RAM for your mind. It consists of all the things you're keeping in your mind simultaneously. ADHDers struggle with this function, so you must find another way to achieve the same results.

Brainstorming, writing all your thoughts down about your life goals and problems, is the key to offsetting this challenge.

First, by writing down your thoughts on a whiteboard or paper, you can hold more ideas than you could in your limited working memory. This means you can more easily work through complex issues while keeping all the information together in one place.

The great advantage of a whiteboard is all your thoughts become a physical visual reality. This helps your brain consider all the possibilities at the same time.

Before you clean the whiteboard, take a photo and save it on your computer for later reference. Your computer becomes your working memory with unlimited storage and instant retrieval.

Second, writing everything down allows you to go back and edit it. You can add additional information and remove ideas that aren't up to standard.

Use colour-coded post-it notes or coloured whiteboard markers to place ideas into a different section of a complex issue so your brain doesn't get confused.

Third, writing allows for longer thoughts. Have you ever had a conversation where, as you were listening, you forgot the point you were eager to make? Ideas pop up all the time in your mind; writing allows you to capture them.

You have created your world and reality with your thoughts. If you want to change your world, you must change your thoughts.

MASTER YOUR THOUGHTS

All self-discipline begins with the mastery of your thoughts. If you don't control what you think, you can't control what you do.

The primary cause of unhappiness is never the situation but your thoughts about it. You have to become constantly aware of what you are thinking.

Your subconscious mind will act on thoughts conveyed with desire backed by positive emotions.

Powered by desire, your subconscious mind will do anything to obtain the object of your desire. It will also open all available channels to the conscious mind for information on how to do it.

When you have set your subconscious mind to the task backed up with intense emotion, it allows you to see the opportunities in life that lead you to your goals.

Ask your subconscious mind to look for opportunities to achieve your goals.

PERFECTION IS BULLSH*T

Everyone falls off the wagon. The difference is the successful ones accept they are human and get back on track quickly without allowing guilt or low self-confidence to control their thoughts and stop their momentum.

Setbacks are to be expected and just like life, are only temporary. You won't be able to get rid of all your painful thoughts, feelings and life circumstances. That's impossible.

The goal is to change your response to them. To be in the midst of 'life' and to be in control mentally, emotionally and physically.

Simply start over. If you drop out on your routine because of work, an unexpected illness or just a sh*t day, don't overthink it – just start again where you left off. You don't have to be perfect every day to achieve your goals and dreams.

Thinking can become addictive, making you feel like you are making progress. However, thought has to be joined by action to gain real value from your efforts of thinking.

SUMMARY

- Think less; do more.
- Thoughts are not facts.
- Think it over. Don't overthink it.
- Clear thinking saves time and energy.
- Learn to master your thoughts, or by default, you allow your thoughts to control you.

ACTIONS

Your thoughts become your things.

HOW TO MASTER YOUR THOUGHTS

1. Accept that awareness and mastering your thoughts are critical to your success and are totally within your control.
2. Constantly fill your mind with empowering thoughts and images aligned with your primary goals and purpose.
3. Erase and replace – when you notice an ANT (automatic negative thought), call up your opposite PET (positive empowering thought) to blow it away.
4. Notice if you start to feel tension or uncertainty and know that your negative inner voice is running on your old, outdated

program. Say thank you for sharing and hit DELETE. Just like you would delete junk email, hit delete! Stop the cycle.
5. If the thoughts are persistent, backtrack and ask yourself what the false beliefs are behind the thoughts. Reaffirm your new beliefs and identity.
6. Remind yourself what outcome or result you want. Stay focused and take immediate action towards your goals and desires. Don't get distracted or overthink the issue.
7. To help take control of your thoughts, build your support systems, like rituals and habits. You could carry a talisman, a lucky charm, a rubber band around your wrist, a ring, or something else you identify with positively. Whenever your thoughts are trending towards the negative, touch your symbol and get them back into the positive.
8. Try this quick breathing exercise if you are struggling to delete limiting thoughts and feel the associated emotions building. Deep breath in for 3 seconds, hold and slowly count to 8, then breathe out fully, visualising your mind releasing the thought and emotions. Do this six times.

YOUR THOUGHTS

NOTES

9

YOUR EMOTIONS & FEELINGS

WHAT'S THE DIFFERENCE?

Emotions are physical and instinctive. They are caused by chemicals subconsciously released by your brain in response to a specific event or trigger.

Feelings form when you consciously or subconsciously assign meaning to the emotional experience you are having. Feelings happen as you begin to consciously think about the emotion, to 'let it soak in'. They are your response or reaction to the emotions.

The fundamental difference between feelings and emotions is that feelings are experienced consciously while emotions happen subconsciously.

ADHD ADDults

Example

Let's say you are home alone at night and hear a loud noise in the kitchen. On a subconscious level, your brain instinctively responds by releasing chemicals into your body and brain that instantly change your mental, physical and emotional states. You will become acutely aware of your surroundings, listening for further noises or movements.

You will start to consciously think about the noise. Your brain will assign a meaning to the emotional event you are experiencing based on your beliefs and life experiences associated with this type of noise.

Thoughts will start to flood your mind. Is someone in the kitchen? Did I leave the window open, and something has blown over? Is the cat on the kitchen bench again? Am I in danger? Should I run away? Your thoughts will produce the corresponding emotions and feelings. It could be fear, annoyance, anxiety, surprise and anything in between.

Don't build a wall around your feelings to avoid pain and misery because you will also block out happiness, joy, excitement and creativity.

EMOTIONS

Your emotions are physical. You can't control them as they are hardwired into your genes over many years of evolution. Their purpose is to produce a specific response to a stimulus.

From an evolutionary standpoint, your emotions help you act, strive, avoid danger, make instant decisions and survive. They power your actions; your fight, flight or freeze response.

You display some emotions outwardly both verbally through words and nonverbally through facial expressions, voice volume and pitch, gestures, body language, and movements.

These displays of emotions serve as social signals that help other people to understand you. They also allow you to interact with others' needs in mind rather than your own, which is the foundation of society.

An event or situation might evoke more than one emotion. You may experience multiple different emotions to varying degrees that make up your emotional cocktail.

In general, people can be terrible at recognising the emotions in themselves and others, which leads to a lot of misunderstandings. Emotions carry information and are open to interpretation. They are not necessarily logical.

Today, emotions remain the first filter for all the information you receive. You know you are supposed to act rationally, but your emotions can never be entirely suppressed.

6 TYPES OF EMOTIONS

| Anger | Disgust | Fear |

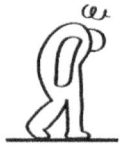

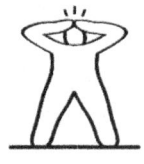

Happiness   Sadness   Surprise

During the 1970s, psychologist Paul Eckman identified six basic emotions he suggested were universally experienced in all human cultures. The emotions he identified were:

Over time, this list of basic emotions has been added to, subtracted from, and reshaped. In 2017 a study expanded it to twenty-seven emotions.(15)

Admiration, adoration, aesthetic, appreciation amusement, anger, anxiety, awe, awkwardness, boredom, calmness, confusion, craving, disgust, entrancement, excitement, fear, horror, interest, joy, nostalgia, relief, romance, sadness, satisfaction, sexual desire, surprise.

Emotions can and sometimes will get the better of you. The goal isn't to suppress these emotions; it is to change your response to them. To be in the midst of 'life' and to be in control mentally, emotionally and physically, and to build emotional resilience.

Positive and negative emotions play a vital role in executive functions: initiating and prioritising tasks, sustaining or shifting interest or effort, and holding thoughts in your active memory.

Look within and pinpoint the situations creating stress and negative emotions in your life. By looking at the source of the feeling and the belief behind your reaction, it can provide valuable insight. Learn some coping strategies to help you respond instead of reacting emotionally to challenging situations.

Example

Let's look at some of the most powerful emotions and how they can impact your life.

FEAR

> *'Fear is the most destructive emotion we can experience. It is caused by ignorance.'*
>
> **Bob Proctor**

While we feel many emotions, one, in particular, bears discussing in depth. Fear.

Fear stems from a real or imagined loss. It is an unpleasant emotion caused by the perception of danger, pain or harm.

It is the most powerful of all emotions and can override even the strongest aspects of your intelligence. Fear is designed to keep you safe, using your fight or flight response. You are hardwired to survive, not thrive.

While fear is essential for your survival, it can also stop you from moving forward in pursuit of your dreams and goals.

But fear in the right doses can be fun and exciting. Many people use fear to scare themselves – deliberately. They run across deserts, ride roller coasters, go skydiving, race cars, drop off mountains or take on massive business challenges.

Fear can make you feel alive. The excitement generated can also help alleviate depression by increasing adrenaline, which in turn increases arousal, excitement, and glucose for energy.

> *When afraid, your brain fires off chemicals. Stress hormones like cortisol and adrenaline are released. Your blood pressure and heart rate increase. Your senses buzz to life. Fear provides energy; use it intelligently. Choose to make fear your ally.*
>
> *ADHDers often seek high-risk activities to get their boost of dopamine. However, too much can be detrimental and make you crash and burn.*
>
> *While being fully engaged and focused on a stimulating activity, the chemical cocktail of natural opioids released from your brain makes the 'noises' in your head fade, and you may feel very calm.*
>
> *That is why you can remain focused and calm in a critical situation or profession. A dose of fear is a 'cleaner' for the mind.*

NAME YOUR FEAR

Fear of failure, success, ridicule, change, guilt.

Fear of who I am, the unknown, of loss, rejection.

Fear of snakes, spiders, heights, flying, water.

Fear of death, dogs, to name a few.

The fear response comes from sensing real or imagined danger. It often leads to a fight-or-flight response. In extreme cases of fear, there may be a freeze response, paralysis, or procrastination.

Don't allow fears to make you question your goals or whether you can achieve success. Never lose sight of your ability to overcome challenges, find solutions, succeed over adversity, and achieve your goals.

Use fear to drive you forward, not to hold you back.

EMOTIONS AND ADHD

People with ADHD feel emotions more intensely. Your emotions can struggle to distinguish between dangerous threats and minor problems. You don't just get happy; you are ecstatic, and when something bad happens, you're *shattered*.

Those with ADHD tend to have less 'bandwidth' in their working memory functions and are likely to have more difficulty than others in quickly linking together various memories relevant to doing or not doing a task. They are less likely to consider the bigger picture of which the present moment is a part.

Thomas Brown, PhD, describes the overwhelming power of emotions often experienced by a person with ADHD as 'flooding'. Emotions can use up all the available space in your brain, and other thoughts or feelings are displaced.

He also mentions that the individual with ADHD has issues shifting from one emotion to another. Therefore, it is possible to 'get stuck' in an emotional state. Brown describes the difficulty that individuals might experience in identifying whether a problem is major or minor, which might result in 'catastrophising it'.

Overwhelming emotions can take over and impede your intentions, making it extremely challenging to accomplish things you truly want or need to do.

The good news is that your brain is adaptable, and you can manage your emotions by being aware of your thoughts and feelings.

First, recognise when emotions are flooding you and manage those emotions. Self-regulation is all about staying in control. This will improve your ability to deal with change and resolve conflict.

Use self-awareness, so you always know how you feel, and you know how your emotions and actions can affect the people around you.

You often feel powerless to control them and can be thrown into panic mode by thoughts or perceptions that cause you to overreact. Your reduced working memory capacity is the issue.

It's usually the reactions that create challenges, not the emotions themselves.

Beware of using self-sabotaging or destructive ways to cope with negative emotions.

FEELINGS

Feelings are emotions processed by thinking, a cognitive process. Because they are based on an individual's experience, feelings can be entirely subjective and vary from person to person.

People or events cannot directly impact your feelings. It is the meaning you attach to an event.

You can control your thoughts, and by changing your thoughts, you can consciously alter your feeling about any situation.

Being able to alter your feelings gives you a great sense of empowerment and personal control.

Never make an important decision based on temporary or volatile feelings.

Your feeling can come from any of the six basic emotions making you happy, sad, frightened, disgusted, angry or surprised.

YOUR EMOTIONS & FEELINGS

Feelings can also come from any of your five senses within your environment, such as warmth, cold, hot, dry, dusty or dirty.

Or they might come from physical sensations like hunger, thirst, pain or exhaustion.

Feelings play out in your head. They are your thoughts and interpretations of an event that are personal and acquired through your life experiences and can influence your thinking processes, sometimes in constructive ways, sometimes not.

It is difficult to think critically and clearly when you have intense feelings.

Feelings are caused by thoughts about circumstances and people. People or circumstances in and of themselves cannot directly impact your feelings. Being crystal clear about this concept will give you a great sense of empowerment and freedom.

The emotion comes first and is universal. What kind of feeling(s) it will then become varies enormously from person to person and from situation to situation because feelings are shaped by individual temperament and experience. Two people can experience the same event but feel differently.

Example

Two people visit a zoo, and they see a gorilla in a beautiful walled area. One feels awe, curiosity and admiration for such a magnificent creature while the other feels bitterness as they believe gorillas should never be held captive.

Because feelings are based on an individual's emotional experience, they can be entirely subjective and vary from person to person.

Feelings form when your brain assigns a meaning to the emotional experience you are having.

How you feel drives your actions or inactions. When you feel good, you're more creative, resourceful and productive. When you are in a positive mindset, you readily take the actions you need to achieve your goals.

FEELINGS AND WORKING MEMORY

Your working memory capacity impacts your ability to deal with pleasant and unpleasant feelings without getting excessively caught up in them.

Working memory is your short-term memory, which is important for reasoning, learning and understanding. It is a 'temporary storage system' in the brain that holds several facts or thoughts while you are solving a problem or performing a task. It is the ability to retain information for short periods while processing or using it.

It helps you hold information long enough to use it in the short term, focus on a task, and remember what to do next. Working memory is essential for keeping in mind the relative priorities of your various interests at any given time.

Sometimes your ADHD-limited working memory allows a temporary emotion to become too strong or lack sensitivity to the importance of a particular emotion because you haven't kept other relevant information in mind.

Some people with ADHD don't suffer from a lack of awareness of important emotions but from an inability to cope with those emotions long enough to deal with them effectively.

*Emotions cannot persist unless you
give them your attention.*

YOUR EMOTIONS & FEELINGS

Working memory brings into play, consciously and/or unconsciously, the emotional energy needed to help us organise, sustain focus, monitor and self-regulate.

A lack of adequate working memory may explain why you can be disorganised, lose your cool or procrastinate. This can lead to low energy, lack of motivation and damaged self-esteem, which play havoc with your emotions.

Emotions drive your actions and behaviours. When you feel good, you're more creative, resourceful and productive. When you're in a positive frame of mind, you readily take the actions needed to achieve your goals.

One function of working memory is to keep track of input. This system evaluates incoming information and keeps attention moving forward. Information is held and evaluated, and a decision is made to discard the information or save it for later use.

Improved working memory allows you to work faster by retaining certain information that you'll soon need to reuse instead of taking additional time to write it down or redo a task because you forget something.

You may operate more like someone watching a basketball game through a telescope, unable to consider the rest of the action on the court, the threats and/or opportunities that are not included in the small circle of focus.(11)

FEELINGS AND MOTIVATION

How you feel is a large part of the driving force behind the motivation that moves you forward or holds you back. You need positive feelings to prepare you to take action; they provide the drive.

Feelings like frustration and boredom can lower motivation and, thus, reduce the chance that you will act.

Sometimes you just don't feel like doing what you are supposed to do. Other times you are motivated.

You can become caught up in behaviour habits to avoid or procrastinate dealing with overwhelming or painful feelings linked to financial, personal or work challenges.

Neuroscience has shown that conscious feelings are only a tiny part of the range of emotions that operates within each person to motivate executive functions.

Be aware of your intellectual and emotional 'state', listen to your feelings, and then change to a positive 'state'.

SUMMARY

- Emotions are what drive you.
- Emotions are physical and primal.
- Feelings are caused by your thoughts about the emotions you are experiencing.
- Controlling your feelings allows you to respond instead of reacting.

Learn how to get yourself into a positive emotional state when you need superior performance.

ACTIONS

1. If you start to feel fear or doubt, write down what you fear. Ask yourself, is it real or imagery?
2. Fear is a result of ignorance. Knowledge and action will crush your fear. Next, make a list of two or three actions you can take to defeat this fear, and take immediate action.

YOUR EMOTIONS & FEELINGS

3. Emotions are what drive you. Learn how to get into a positive emotional state for learning, creating and when you need superior performance. Change your physiology, do some form of physical movement, sit or stand upright, walk the stairs or go outside, breathe deeply, feel the positive energy rising from your feet to your head.
4. Practice emotional awareness and regulate your feelings by using meditation, journaling, listening to music, watching, reading, or listening to something inspiring. If you are really struggling seek help. Ask your ADHD ADDults community for advice or talk to an ADHD coach. Do what feels right for you.
5. Get restful sleep. Make sure you're consistent with your sleep and waking times, and optimise your bedroom environment. Don't drink alcohol or excessive amounts of caffeine. Supply your body and ADHD brain with top-quality fuel.
6. Get regular exercise to get the oxygen pumping through your body and brain. It lowers your body's stress hormones, such as adrenaline and cortisol. Exercise also stimulates the production of endorphins, chemicals in the brain that are the body's natural painkillers and mood elevators.(16)

Your emotions and feelings drive your behaviour.

NOTES

10

YOUR BEHAVIOUR

Your behaviour, both conscious and subconscious, is how you respond to internal and external events in your life. It is also influenced by your unique personality traits, beliefs, values, thoughts and feelings.

Thoughts and feelings are internal aspects that you don't have to act on. By contrast, your behaviour is what you do, how you act in the world.

Feelings vary. One minute, you're happy, then something happens that makes you angry or frustrated. Your ADHD makes your feelings much more intense, and this clouds your judgment and response.

Sometimes when you are frustrated, you say and do things that you're not proud of. How you feel directly impacts your behaviour.

Your behaviour is a combination of your routines, rituals and habits.

```
       Routines
          |
      BEHAVIOUR
       /     \
   Rituals   Habits
```

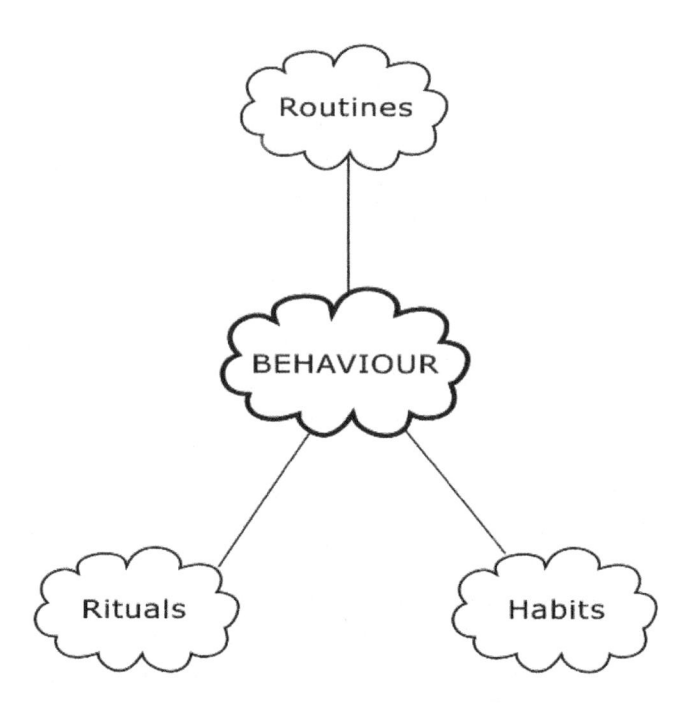

WHAT'S THE DIFFERENCE?

Behaviours that require concentration, deliberation or extended effort are not habits.

Routines are a set of behaviours in a particular order that you do with some frequency but not automatically. Routines don't care if you feel an urge or not; they just need to get done like buying food, putting fuel in the car, doing the washing, feeding the dogs or taking a shower.

A ritual is a carefully selected way of doing something with a sense of purpose. The intent is that the ritual has a specific purpose that will help you achieve an important goal or dream. For me, one is going to the gym. I train with the purpose of being as mentally and physically fit as I can.

A habit is a learned behaviour you do automatically without thinking about it, something you do repeatedly and perform subconsciously. It might be driving, brushing your teeth or walking the dog.

ROUTINES

A routine is a series of behaviours you practice regularly.

It's important to recognise that not all routines can become habits. Some actions will remain routines and require effort and discipline.

Expect that learning and repeatedly doing a new behaviour will require effort. Expect some discomfort and know that you'll have to push through it.

Your daily routine provides structure and a logical sequence in your life. It provides the framework within which you live your life and conduct daily activities. You become familiar and comfortable with what you have to do each day. It allows you to experience flow in your day.

Routine can be helpful when it comes to managing your busy life. It can help you fit all of the essential things into your day. The predictability of routine can offer some certainty in an otherwise unpredictable world.

Structured routines allow you to set aside blocks of time for important things that are a necessary part of your daily physical and mental health.

Focus on forming structured patterns and use mini rewards as a way to stick to your routines.

Carefully designing a set routine to follow eliminates indecision and the need to plan your activities every morning.

It gives structure to your day and allows you to wake up and *do* instead of wake up and *plan*, saving you precious time and energy.

Over time some routines become your habits.

RITUALS

The difference between a daily routine and a daily ritual is knowing the intended purpose behind the ritual.

Rituals are thoughtful actions with a sense of purpose – like meditation. Rituals have always existed in society, and you already have some of your own rituals.

There's a balance to be found between routine and ritual. We'll always have routines that we need to do to be efficient. There's always stuff that simply needs to be done.

But there's a lot of value in finding routines (or even parts of routines) that we can turn into rituals for the benefit of a better day.

Rituals can help you take the boredom or stress out of regular activity. They can help you be more thoughtful, connect to your purpose and achieve your goals.

The familiar structure of a ritual will help your ADHD brain to feel a sense of control, calm your anxiety and increase your confidence. A daily ritual can provide energy and enjoyment along with efficiency.

This will add more meaning because you understand how your routines are helping you to achieve a bigger purpose.

You already have daily routines. You can transform some of those routines into positive daily rituals with the right attitude. These rituals help you focus, feel motivated, inspired and achieve your goals.

Pick one of your routines and think about how you can turn it from a mundane autopilot task to a more meaningful experience in your day.

> **Example**
>
> *For me, I get everything ready in the evening that I will need to get my next day off to a great start. Clothes, food, paperwork, and my morning rituals gear. The purpose or intent is to give me a structured start to my day and I don't have to think for the first thirty minutes after my feet hit the floor.*

You are a unique individual with your own purpose and set of goals that you want to achieve. There's no right or wrong set of rituals to follow. The secret to success is identifying your daily routines that can be turned into the rituals that inspire and motivate you to achieve your set of goals.

> *Rituals are a cornerstone of the foundations upon which your success will be built.*

HABITS

> *Your brain doesn't recognise habits as good or bad.*

Routines and rituals are done consciously, while a habit is done unconsciously. If you are unconsciously repeatedly reacting to a given situation, it has become a habit. If it isn't making your life better, you need to change.

Everything you do subconsciously is a learned habit; it is not thinking. They can be empowering or disempowering, but everything you do without thinking is a habit.

Human nature follows the law of minimum effort. You will naturally gravitate towards the option that requires the least amount of work.

Habits are shortcuts to help your mind conserve energy. You are neurologically designed to seek organisation and patterns in the environment and actions, using predictable and familiar patterns to navigate the day on 'autopilot'.

Then, your best attention, effort and energy are available for dealing with new and unfamiliar events and experiences.

YOUR HABITS

Your habits determine what actions you take consistently.

Break your habits into three groups.

1. The first group is the habits that we simply overlook because they have been part of our lives forever – like riding a bike, washing your hair or brushing your teeth.
2. The second are habits that are good for you and that you work hard on establishing – like exercising, eating well or getting enough sleep.
3. The final group is negative habits like smoking, procrastinating or overspending.

You created an unhealthy habit to help you deal with stress or anxiety about a situation that was resolved ages ago, but the habit remains though it serves no purpose.

Your life today is essentially the sum of your routines, rituals and habits. How healthy, happy and prosperous you are is a direct result.

Every habit produces some benefit, a reward for your brain even if it's bad for you, like smoking.

YOUR BEHAVIOUR

Habits are repeated actions that have become automatic and may be harder to stop.

CHOOSE BETTER HABITS

Your habits can make or break you.

Researchers from Duke University have shown that over 40 per cent of what you do is determined not by decisions but by habits. This suggests that you can change a huge part of your life by eliminating bad habits and creating good ones instead.

The real problem is some of the destructive habits you have developed aren't so obvious.

Because so many of your habits run without conscious control, making habit changes has to start with awareness of your behaviour.

Awareness is knowledge of a situation or fact. The biggest benefit to self-awareness is that it allows you the freedom to choose better routines, rituals and habits, ones that are aligned with your goals and dreams.

We have unhealthy habits for a reason; there's usually a benefit. Identify the benefit and then compensate for the loss of it. If you're going to cut out junk food, for example, identify the reasons why you consume it.

Instead of eating chocolate in the evening because you're sitting in front of the TV, change it to a piece of fruit and some nuts. Retrain your brain to release dopamine from healthy sources.

Chose new habits that have a high return on effort.

CHANGING YOUR HABITS

How long does it take to form a new habit? I have the exact answer – one to three hundred days. Seriously, if you are concerned about how long it will take, you need to rethink the whole concept.

It doesn't matter how long it takes. What matters is the benefits the new habit will bring into your life. If you plan on using willpower: ditto.

Use your imagination of the positive benefits to pull you towards building the new habit instead of pushing through the pain. It's about mindset and the vision you hold in your head.

It all comes back to your beliefs and identity.

Your behaviour is a reflection of your current identity.

Your habits are how you express your beliefs.

Habits are a two-sided coin. They can stop you from achieving the life you want or provide you with the life you want.

Each habit, the good, the bad or the ugly, reinforces your beliefs and subsequent identity.

Look at your beliefs and identity to help you change any habit that isn't supporting you, your goals and your life's purpose.

Make dramatic changes to your physical and mental environment if that is what it takes.

⚠️

Yes, you can. That is only fear and excuses trying to keep you where you are. Say thank you for sharing, and hit the DELETE button.

YOUR BEHAVIOUR

To change your eating habits, change your routines, such as where you buy your food and what you buy.

Look for new and more nutritious food from different sources. It is easier to remove the temptation than to use willpower.

IMPULSE CONTROL AND DELAYED REWARDS

One of your major challenges is to learn to delay short-term gratification to allow for greater future success.

Impulse control is a skill that you can develop. The reward is on the other side of sacrifice. The athlete's high only comes after the workout.

Self-discipline requires you to release some desires rather than satisfy them.

> *Discipline is the bridge between setting and achieving your goals.*

Eat the apple instead of the doughnut. Save some of your money instead of wasting it.

Your ADHD brain already has a shortage of dopamine and often uses any means to get it that may not be beneficial in the pursuit of your major long-term goals.

There are ways to overcome this tendency for instant rewards. While some discipline is helpful, it's not always the most effective method.

Impulse control is letting go of the desire rather than fulfilling it – try some of these strategies:

- Set a timer on your phone and delay the reward for ten minutes.

- Delaying something can be *the reward*.
- Don't buy it today. Decide to wait until tomorrow to see if it's still life-threatening that you must buy this item.
- Go over your goals. Is it on your list?
- Use awareness to dig into the thoughts behind the desire. Is it cause by stress or boredom?
- Practice controlling your thoughts by thinking of a healthy or better alternative action.
- Think you are hungry? Drink a large glass of water, and wait.
- Be grateful for what you already have while striving for what you want.
- Train your brain to accept a larger reward later on rather than taking the immediate reward.
- Refocus on your major goals and dreams.
- Remind yourself to live on purpose.

Delaying gratification is a strategy for achieving success and long-term fulfilment.

For ADHDers, goal achievement needs to be structured to provide regular mini dopamine feel-good rewards, so you can enjoy the journey by sticking to your systems and working through the processes each day on the way to your goals.

You need to feel you are continually improving, even if it is only in small steps. They will compound over the weeks, months and years ahead.

You will see you are getting closer each time you complete a task and reward yourself with something positive and aligned with your values and lifestyle.

YOUR BEHAVIOUR

Mini rewards help you go the distance.

⚠️

Even with your new rituals, routines and habits, you will still have the occasional rough day when the sh*t hits the fan. Your energy is low and your thoughts are far from positive. You need to be able to take back control of your mindset or 'state'.

Example

Something didn't work out the way you planned and expected. Reality doesn't match your expectations.
Your racing thoughts and negative self-talk go into overdrive. It is disturbing and borders on being destructive.

You don't believe you can do what it takes to achieve the goals to become the person in your dreams. You lose your confidence, which then makes everything seem even worse. You can feel the rising tide of being overwhelmed.

Phase 1

STOP what you are doing, recognise and accept you are feeling like sh*t, and defuse your self-sabotaging behaviour by doing the following:

- *Change your physiology, stand or sit upright, hold your head high and slap your chest or leg and say to yourself or aloud, 'I am capable, I am worthy, I am enough!'*

- *Don't make any major decisions or speak what is on your mind from this unstable emotional mindset.*
- *Don't ask anyone for their opinion.*
- *Challenge all non-supporting thoughts and replace them with positive, empowering thoughts (PETs).*
- *Stop any non-supporting beliefs, thoughts, or actions.*

Phase 2

Now reset your subconscious mind by thinking intently of positive and inspiring thoughts with your conscious mind.

- *Isolate yourself, and get some quiet solo time. (Go and sit on a toilet if you have to.)*
- *Take 6 or 7 deep breaths, in through your nose, out through your mouth. (Wim Hof style.)*
- *Relax your body.*
- *Release all the tension.*
- *Still your mind.*
- *Be grateful for everything you have now while pursuing what you want.*
- *Feel your powerful positive energy returning.*
- *See and feel as you would when you have already achieved your goals.*
- *Take some form of immediate action towards your goals.*

SUMMARY

- Routines are conscious actions that just need to be done.
- Rituals are actions with a sense of purpose.
- A habit is an action you do automatically without having to think about it.

- Both good and bad habits are dopamine-seeking behaviours. Choose good ones and DELETE the bad ones.
- Make your new habits simple to do and enjoyable.

ACTIONS

1. Look at your current primary goals and identify a few key supportive routines, rituals or habits that will be the most helpful in reaching your specific goals.

    - Say you want to stay in a more positive headspace so you can invest more time and energy in pursuing your goals. You could develop a ritual of feeding your mind and body positive energy by listening to empowering media while doing some form of physical activity.

2. Pick 1 or 2 things you do every day that you could add intention and purpose to and make into a daily ritual?

    - Let's say you have a 30-minute daily work commute. Use that time to listen to empowering podcasts, videos or audiobooks to improve your knowledge or maybe find a solution to a problem.

3. Pick a habit you want to adopt and then do it just for today, for 14 days. It's just 14 days. Anybody can do something for 14 days. Then review, adjust and repeat.

4. Control how you manage your environment in your busy life. Get into the habit of setting your work area up to be ADHD-friendly.

    - Start by removing any visual distractions. That includes any distracting screen backgrounds, keeping it a single colour of your choice, putting everything into folders, and putting all those folders in ONE main folder on your screen. When working on your primary task, you only take out the folders you need to get the job done. There are no other distractions on your screen.

Example

When I am working on a multiple-page word document and get distracted by the other information on the page, I copy and paste only the text I want to work on and put it on a fresh page to help me focus better. When I am finished, I copy and paste it back onto the main document and hit save!

---

5. Remove external distractions.

- Turn your phone to aeroplane mode. Close down your emails. Isolate yourself if you can. If not physically, then learn to do it mentally. Close the door, or wear a headset or earbuds to restrict outside distractions.

6. If you want to learn more about habits, check out the likes of BJ Fogg, Charles Duhigg, and James Clear, but in the end, you need to design the routines, rituals and habits that will work best for your ADHD brain.

YOUR BEHAVIOUR

NOTES

11

YOUR ACTIONS

Your actions determine your results.

You are designed to be physically and mentally active. Your actions are a vital part of the fabric of your life and produce all your results.

Your best intentions and ideas will amount to nothing without consistent, deliberate and intelligent action. Without action, it's all only a dream.

What you believe, and your skills, talents and knowledge are wasted if you don't take action.

The universe only rewards action.

Action inspires, and consistent action has a cumulative effect, building self-confidence and the desire to take even more action. But you must start!

Taking action also quiets your significant other, *your inner voice*. You know the one that says, you're stupid; you're useless; no, that will never work; you could never do that.

Every time you do something new, you expand your comfort zone just a bit. And, as you expand your comfort zone, you are more willing to come out of your corner and do things that benefit your life.

The benefits of consistently taking massive action are:

- Creates momentum
- Creates a ripple effect previously unseen
- Opens up new pathways and possibilities
- Provides the opportunity to get real value from the time and effort you invested in learning and acquiring knowledge
- Expands your knowledge, awareness and understanding of the world around you
- Allows you to make mistakes faster, to learn and adjust and get better
- Teaches you new skills and expands your brain's ability
- Introduces different people and exciting and unexpected experiences into your life
- Defeats procrastination
- It becomes a habit

CAUSE AND EFFECT

The universal law of cause and effect is very simple and very obvious. Successes, as well as failures, are not accidents. Every result, single solitary success or failure, can be traced back to a specific action or inaction.

This law of *cause and effect* states that for every cause (action), there is a definite effect (result).

YOUR ACTIONS

Your thoughts, behaviours and actions cause specific effects that manifest and create your life as you know it.

Cause is the reason something happened.

Effect is the result of what happened.

Example

The cause is eating too much food without any physical activity. The effect is you will gain weight.

A wild storm blew the roof off the house, and as a result, the family has to find another place to live.

If you are not happy with the effects you have created, then you must change the causes that created them in the first place ... your actions or inactions.

For every effect in your life, there is a specific cause.

Therefore, you can trace the effect all the way back to the cause. If we keep repeating the same cause (your actions), we should expect to get more of the same effects (your results). Only when you decide to change your actions can you expect new and different results.

Your actions show the world your true intentions.

WHAT'S THE COST OF INACTION?

Inaction can lead to many negative consequences in your life. They may not appear in the first few days or a week or month, but you reap what you sow, and sooner or later, they will show up.

These negative impacts can affect your physical and mental health, finances, career, and relationships, especially the one with yourself!

Not taking action results in mental and physical pain. The regret of not doing what you want, the lack of growth and confidence in yourself, and the negative self-talk all result in unnecessary mental pain.

Don't underestimate the damage inaction causes. Every day you choose inaction over action makes it harder to take action.

Lack of action causes the following effects:

- Boredom – very dangerous for ADHDers
- Opens the doorway to fear and doubts
- Confusion
- Indecision and uncertainty
- Kills momentum
- Kills your dreams
- Shuts the door to opportunity
- Wastes your precious time
- Shuts down motivation
- Lowers self-belief
- Derails achievement
- Feeds mental health issues

The only time inaction has any value is when you plan to use it for your benefit in any of the following ways:

- Quiet solo time
- Meditation
- Rest and recovery

- Personal reflection
- Seeking serenity
- Quality sleep

MAJOR CAUSES OF INACTION

Fear: many fears are an illusion created in your mind. It is what causes feelings of anxiety, procrastination, avoidance, worry, anxiousness, suspicion, doubt, agitation, anger and distraction.

Fear, which is almost always the result of destructive self-talk, is based on things that haven't happened and in over 90 per cent of cases don't happen.

Your false and limiting beliefs feed your fears and provide you with excuses to justify your inaction. Inaction leads to a lack of self-confidence in your ability.

You form a never-ending loop of inaction.

You don't want to pay the price of effort or pain.

> *'We must all suffer from one of two pains: the pain of discipline or the pain of regret. The difference is discipline weighs ounces while regret weighs tons.'*
>
> **Jim Rohn**

PROCRASTINATION

The cost of procrastination is catastrophic.

Procrastination is when you delay a required task or action, despite knowing it is harmful to achieving your goals.

So why do you procrastinate?

A major benefit of procrastination is that by not starting on a task or goal, you can't fail, so you can live forever with the fantasy of your future potential.

ADHDers can be perfectionists who are often procrastinators; it is psychologically more acceptable to never start a task than to face the possibility of falling short on ability and performance.

Procrastination can be caused by the size of the task, which makes taking action more difficult.

Procrastination, in large part, reflects your struggles with uncertainty, as well as your inability to predict how you'll feel tomorrow or the day after. 'I don't feel like it' takes precedence over your goals.

Sometimes your brain uses procrastination as a tool. It's an involuntary, subconscious protection trigger to help you avoid dealing with a potentially painful or uncomfortable experience. It's an emotional issue you are avoiding.

Just think about all the time you've spent NOT doing the things that were most important, most profitable and most beneficial for you. Procrastination is a major issue and brings severe consequences.

What's the real cost of your procrastination?

To make it easier to get started, decide to work on a task for only five minutes and see what happens. Remove any pressure or desire to perform well and permit yourself to do a poor job. To get into 'flow' you have to start.

> *Don't confuse preparation with action. Preparation and action are not the same things. Don't get bogged down in the analysing, planning, organising and preparation stages when you need to take action.*

Example

I research articles to help me lose body fat by altering my nutrition and decide to cut back my portion sizes by 10 per cent. That is preparation.

I have the morning meal, and I reduced my natural Greek yogurt from 170 grams to 150 grams. I reduced the blueberries and the whey protein by 10 per cent. That is action.

DISTRACTIONS

Everyone puts things off sometimes, but ADHDers chronically avoid difficult tasks and deliberately look for distractions.

When you're so distracted by outside stimuli and internal thoughts, it can be hard to get started on a task, especially if that task is difficult or not interesting to you.

> *Overcoming fear, procrastination, and distractions requires self-awareness and self-discipline.*

SUMMARY

- Inaction kills dreams.
- Action is the vaccine for fear.
- Only your actions produce results.
- The universal law of cause and effect is absolute.
- Action is the only way you can turn your dreams into physical reality.

ACTIONS

1. Look at one of your major goals and write down three concrete steps you can take over the 30 days that will move you closer to achieving the goal. Next, write a list of tasks, big or small, then for the next 30 days, work on those tasks every day whether you feel like it or not. It will build momentum, and you will start to see opportunities that were not visible before.
2. Start to become more aware of how the law of cause and effect impacts your life. Look for an area of your life that you're not happy with and find the cause so you can change your actions. It may not be dramatic but something simple.
3. Defeat inaction by knowing the high cost of sitting on the fence. What fears are stopping you from taking action? Decide what is the worst that can happen, then take action to reduce the likelihood of it occurring.
4. Seeking perfection, not knowing where to start, and feeling overwhelmed are major causes of procrastination. How do you eat an elephant? One bite at a time. Who cares where you start? Just start and adjust as you move forward.
5. Distraction is anything you use to stop you from taking action. Take control of your mind. Ask, 'Is this distraction moving me closer to or further away from the goals I chose?' Change your behaviour accordingly.

NOTES

12

7 KEY ELEMENTS FOR ACTION

Taking constant action will inspire you and has a compounding effect; do something every day towards your major life goal ... every day. It doesn't have to be instantly life-changing, but over time it will become life-changing.

1. ENERGY

To take massive action, you need to generate massive energy.

You need mental and physical energy to first survive and then thrive.

Energy, like time, can't be saved.

You need:

- Physical energy to do what is necessary
- Emotional energy to enjoy your life
- Mental energy to learn and make better decisions
- Spiritual energy to contribute and feel fulfilled

Let's say you start each day with one hundred energy credits to spend as you see fit. With shifting priorities, how you spend them might vary day-to-day. You must allocate your energy in the right areas on the right things.

Your energy levels will vary throughout the day, and it's important to match your energy to the task for the best possible outcomes.

You also need to recognise when you don't have sufficient mental or emotional energy to make major decisions. Reschedule them so that your energy levels match the task.

You generate a certain amount of energy each day. This will vary from person to person and day-to-day. Your physical health, daily nutrition, sleep, mental attitude, beliefs and actions all impact your energy levels.

Your brain doesn't store energy. Unlike muscles, which can store excess carbohydrates, the brain needs to be constantly supplied with oxygen and energy to run properly and support and sustain your life.

Mentally challenging activities, such as work, hobbies, reading and studying, require energy. According to the Franklin Institute, brain cells require twice as much energy needed by other cells.

You also need quality sleep. It is essential for the recovery of your body and mind after a long day. Poor sleep is the major cause of low energy levels and poor executive function and productivity.

7 KEY ELEMENTS FOR ACTION

You cannot run a Ferrari brain on cheap fuel.

You need the right fuel at the right time to maintain optimum energy levels. Never let your tank get empty. It is important to maintain stable blood sugar levels.

Overeating can be just as bad as starvation. The challenge is to be prepared and carry healthful snacks with you so that you don't go for long periods without quality fuel.

If you are active, your energy needs are greater than someone who leads a sedentary lifestyle.

Worry and stress drain mental and physical energy. According to Purdue University Student Health Centre, low energy increases susceptibility to illness.

For the average adult in a resting state, the brain consumes about 20 per cent of the body's energy. Your brain never shuts off. Even when you're sleeping at night, the brain consumes roughly as much energy as it does during the day.(12)

Your brain has sixty litres of blood pumped through it every hour, providing oxygen and nutrients, and removing waste products.(12) If your blood is nutrient-deficient, it will interfere with your brain's ability to create necessary neurotransmitters, which is already an issue in your ADD brain.

You must give your brain the best possible fuel.

To give yourself some downtime during the day, try meditation or deep breathing. Put on some headphones and listen to soothing music for ten minutes with your eyes closed to recharge the body and brain.

You are what you eat. Bad food like processed carbs, refined sugars and synthetic oils creates inflammation within your body and damages your gut lining. This will kill your mood and energy levels.

Instead of that usual energy dip in the mid-afternoon, try taking a few minutes to close your eyes and jump-start your brain power.

Refuel your dopamine level throughout the day using regular small positive rewards, affirmations, goal visualisation, solo thinking time, and exercise.

SUMMARY

- Energy can't be saved. Invest it wisely.
- The better your fuel, the better your performance.
- Regular exercise increases your energy.
- Meditation increases energy levels.

ACTIONS

1. Exercise almost guarantees that you'll sleep more soundly. It also gives your cells more energy to burn and circulates oxygen. And exercising can lead to higher brain dopamine levels, which helps elevate mood.(9)
2. Stress-induced emotions consume huge amounts of energy. Talking through your issues with a friend, joining an ADHD support group, or finding an ADHD specialist can help diffuse stress. Meditation or music can calm emotions and are also effective tools for reducing stress.(9)
3. Eat for energy. Eat foods with a low glycemic index such as whole grains, high-fibre vegetables, nuts, and healthy coconut or olive oil. In general, high-carbohydrate foods have the highest glycemic indexes. Cut out sugar. Proteins and fats have glycemic indexes that are close to zero.(9)
4. Drink water. If your body is short of fluids, one of the first signs is a feeling of fatigue and brain fog.

7 KEY ELEMENTS FOR ACTION

*When you have your health, you can have
a hundred dreams.
When you don't have your health, you only have
one dream.*

2. TIME

You either invest or waste your precious time.

Time is your most limited and precious resource; you must learn to use it well. As Jim Rohn, a renowned motivational speaker, author, entrepreneur, and business coach, said, 'Most people spend major time on minor things'. Make sure you aren't one of them. You get to choose if you invest or waste your time.

Time to focus on achieving our goals and dreams and fully enjoy those achievements. Time with our families and friends. Time to make a positive impact in the world.

Remember, no one is guaranteed tomorrow, next week or next year. It's best to start investing your time today.

If you tend to read and contemplate a lot and think that the next thing will be the magic pill that will finally solve your problems, you are wasting time. Your life is not endless. Your time is one of the most important things in your life. Don't waste a huge chunk of it.

ADHD ADDults

Start taking action towards what you really want out of life today. You don't want to look back a week, a month or a year from now and wish you had started today.

If you read a non-fiction book and don't act on any of its suggestions, you've wasted time. When reading, always think about how you can apply the teachings in your own life. Study with intent. It's not about how fast you can finish the book so you can start on another one.

Now that you have decided who you want to become, what you want to do and what you want to have, it's best to start right away.

Reaffirm the major projects you want to invest your time in over the next three, six and twelve months.

There are three stages of time – the past, the present and the future. You can use the past to learn and prepare for the future, but the present is the only space where you can take action.

You may spend a lot of time dragging up the past or worrying about the future. If you can't learn from it, let go of the past and look ahead to the future with hope instead of fear. You will feel a lot happier and calmer.

While everyone does technically have twenty-four hours in a day, our amount of *free* time varies dramatically. While someone with a good job with normal working hours can spend a fair amount of time practising a skill, someone who needs to work many more hours to earn the same amount can't. In that sense, even though they both have twenty-four hours in a day, time is relative for them.

Be selective with who you invest your time;
wasted time is worse than wasted money.

When you are committed to your success, it will automatically reflect in how you use your time.

Continuous daily actions and a burning desire towards your goals will help you avoid wasting your time.

One of the dangers of poor time usage is that it kills your chances of broadening your horizons and trying out new things. You miss out on the chance to explore different opportunities.

Don't waste time waiting. Plan in advance so you can use waiting time wisely and to your advantage. Always have a book or media device with you or do some type of exercise instead of getting stressed over lost time.

> *Know the true value of your time; snatch, seize, and enjoy every moment of it.*

3. DELEGATE

> *'Every major success I've had in my life has come about because I knew that somebody, often anybody, whether it was my wife, friend, or business partner, could do something better than I could.'*
>
> **Paul Orfalea, Kinko's**

Delegating and outsourcing are real time savers, which means you have more time to spend on more important tasks while doing less work. Time invested in learning to delegate effectively will repay the initial investment many times over.

Figure out what works best for you if you're struggling with efficient use of your time. The solution may be as simple as changing your schedule around or delegating.

Allow for lag time. It is the time between believing, seeing and feeling something in your conscious mind and its appearance in physical form.

Lag time will vary depending on the size of the dream or goal. Creating your new reality is a process; remain disciplined and committed.

Don't let your mind try and talk you out of it by saying, 'This isn't happening. Let's dump it'. Cultivate patience for larger, longer-term projects. Set up rewards along the way to help you stay in the game long enough to succeed.

Be committed to controlling your time. To succeed in your professional and personal life, you need to eliminate all wasteful activities that don't support you.

Help others, but you aren't everyone's saviour. Don't be afraid or feel guilty about saying no.

The time you have is finite, but the number of choices you have is infinite. Therefore, it is vital to decide precisely how to make the most of the limited time available.

Goals give time direction and purpose.

SUMMARY

- Time is your most valuable asset and resource.
- Delegate and outsource to leverage other people's time.
- Invest quality time with quality people.
- You are going to die; get moving.
- Master your use of time.

ACTIONS

1. Structure your time, even your free time. It will make you more motivated, focused and ultimately happier because it gives you a direction and a purpose for each precious day.
2. For the best use of your time, you need to schedule your 3 to 5 biggest priorities every day.
3. Say 'no' to commitments that don't move you towards your goals and desires.
4. Do less trivial things, and you will be able to invest more of your time into everything important to you.

4. DISCIPLINE

> *'Discipline is doing something you might not like to achieve something you love.'*
>
> **Unknown**

Many of us were raised with false shame-based perceptions of discipline – this involved punishment for being 'bad' and we may have felt judged or rejected.

Self-discipline is a form of freedom. Freedom from laziness and lethargy, freedom from the expectations and demands of others, freedom from weakness and fear or doubt.

Self-discipline, like training or eating, must be done daily. It means self-control, self-mastery and the ability to have 'dinner before dessert'.

Whenever you discipline yourself to do the right thing, whether you feel like it or not, you build respect for yourself. Your self-esteem and self-confidence increase.

You get a payoff every time you hold the line. Your brain releases dopamine.

The only purpose of building self-discipline is to master yourself – your urges, weaknesses and self-sabotaging behaviours.

Discipline is choosing between what you want now and what you want most. It boils down to choosing between instant and delayed gratification. Instant gratification feels good today but compromises your long-term goals.

Delayed gratification usually doesn't deliver much in the short term, but it can lead to bigger rewards in the future.

Self-discipline is about honouring commitments and promises to yourself and others.

Self-discipline is essential to getting things done. We live in a world full of distractions. Self-discipline helps you to focus on your goals by providing order and structure.

Self-discipline is one of the first habits you need to develop. It begins with the mastery of your thoughts. If you don't control what you think, you can't control what you do.

While becoming more self-disciplined is not easy, it's doable. It builds your belief in your ability to do whatever it takes to achieve your objectives.

Seek a disciplined lifestyle for all areas of your life, your health, your business, your career and finances, your relationships, and your personal development.

The unwritten law of discipline:

> *Little bits of discipline achieve little things.*
> *Lots of discipline achieve lots of things.*

7 KEY ELEMENTS FOR ACTION

Discipline your ADHD mind to play the long game by delaying gratification. The principles of life and the laws of the universe never change. They are ageless, constant and absolute.

Discipline is the road that takes you from setting goals to achieving goals.

SUMMARY

- Discipline is a choice.
- Discipline is the path to freedom.
- Self-discipline builds self-confidence.
- Self-discipline is the first stage of self-mastery.

ACTIONS

1. You are wired differently, so approach discipline with an open mind and modify how you achieve the discipline you need to reach your goals. Maybe look at outsourcing your weaker areas rather than trying to master them. Use discipline to build your strengths and manage your challenges.
2. Think self-care over self-indulgence. Using discipline to change your behaviour works best with positive intent. Look at the benefits of the new behaviour, not what you think you are losing. For example, if you change your nutrition and exercise regularly, some of the benefits could be:

    - Improved heart health
    - Better mental performance
    - Greater physical performance
    - Support wealth creation
    - Enjoy your wealth
    - Body fat loss
    - Better tissue and gut health
    - Reduced inflammation
    - Lower cholesterol
    - Boosted executive function

- Detoxification
- Reduced cardiovascular issues
- Increased longevity, vitality and mobility

3. Start early and get some quick wins to build motivation and momentum. Do your most important 3 to 5 tasks first, when your physical and mental energy is highest, and before life gets in the way.
4. Work on continuously improving your physical, mental and emotional environment, so it supports your self-development ambitions. Remove temptations and clutter.

5. DECISIONS

Base every decision on two criteria:

- Does this decision align with my life's purpose?
- Does this decision move me closer to my goals?

You waste time and energy constantly going over the same decisions. To make matters worse, you may enjoy the process of coming up with a never-ending range of choices.

Dopamine is released during the exciting phase of creating multiple solutions, not during the execution. You would rather keep coming up with unlimited possibilities than select only one and have to dump the others.

Because you can see so many options, you end up confused and then don't make any decision. Your life goes on hold until you have to make a decision or the decision is made for you by outside events.

☺

I have trouble deciding because I can see three sides of the coin.

7 KEY ELEMENTS FOR ACTION

Decision-making is a process of reaching a conclusion after careful consideration; it is a judgment, a choice between alternatives when all the facts can't be fully known.

People with ADHD tend towards indecision. Telling someone with ADHD to *just do it* would be like saying *cheer up* to a clinically depressed person.

Decision-making is a key skill you must develop to succeed in life. It is a major task of executive function that you can learn and put structure and templates in place to help you through the process.

ADDers see many options and choices, which can be both a blessing and a curse. Today there is a huge array of choices in your daily life, to the point where it can become detrimental to your life.

Choice means freedom, or does it?

Freedom of choice can be a double-edged sword. To say yes to one thing means saying no to many other bright shiny objects. This can make the process harder and more confusing leading to indecision and procrastination.

True freedom of choice allows you to select an action from at least two available options, unaffected by external influences.

Freedom means being able to compare the situations – the benefits and the drawbacks – and choosing what is best for you. We all desire freedom because, ultimately, freedom brings happiness.

Your daily decisions have a compounding effect on how your life turns out. Should you eat the muffin or the apple? Will you exercise today or watch TV? Will you make that important decision or procrastinate? How will you invest or waste your time today?

Setting priorities helps you to avoid becoming overwhelmed when you have multiple goals you are trying to reach.

Qualify your priorities by answering these questions:

- Will this task move me closer to or further away from my goal?
- Is it really important?
- When will I do this task?
- Where will I do this task
- How will I do this task?

Once you're clear on your priorities, you'll be able to make better and quicker decisions to guide your life choices.

Priorities establish a hierarchy that can be followed for different areas of your life and/or work. Knowing your life's major goals will help you decide how you prioritise your day-to-day tasks.

Certain things are beyond your control: the behaviour of others, your genetics, the weather, gravity, and certain situations. Life can be exciting, messy, challenging and unpredictable at times.

However, you still get to decide what meaning you give these events, how they impact your life, and what you can learn and change. You always have the freedom to choose how you respond.

The quality of your decisions will determine your progress.

Better decisions equal a better life.

Watch the gap between decision and action. Most people don't act as quickly as they should on things. The time to act is when the idea is hot and the emotion is strong.

Decisions, once made, need to be acted on immediately before life blows away the opportunities.

> *The Law of Diminishing Intent*
> *'The longer you wait to do something you should do now, the greater the odds that you will never actually do it.'*
>
> **Jim Rohn**

Make your major decisions based on the highest possibility of success, *not perfection*. This helps to defeat procrastination.

Simplify the process by following the 80/20 rule. Eighty per cent of your decisions are minor decisions and should be solved quickly and without a lot of reflection or overthinking. Twenty per cent are your major decisions, and you need to set aside quiet solo time to think.

Write it down on paper or a whiteboard, *not digitally*. You take the process out of your mind and away from your emotions by putting it on paper. This will help get a better perspective on the issue. Identify the possible effects your choice could have in your life.

Think about and acknowledge the short, medium and long-term consequences, not just the *now* rewards.

Get clear on what you want. What exact outcome do you expect from making this decision? If there are multiple options, use your hierarchy of values to help refine your decision.

- Learned decisiveness is a way of living; without it, you waste precious time and energy.
- Decisions are necessary before actions happen.
- Saying no will make you a better decision maker.
- Learn to be decisive.

Decisions are about freedom of choice, which can be a double-edged sword for ADHDers ... so many bright shiny objects to pick from! To select your goals, you will have to make some decisions about how you want your life to turn out.

It also means saying NO to the unlimited ideas and opportunities your ADHD mind can produce. As they say, you can have anything you want. You just can't have everything. At least not at the same time.

The quality of your decisions determines the quality of your life. First, you must decide what you want your life to be about, the goals and experiences you desire. Making decisions is about defeating fear and procrastination.

Decisions based on your values and current purpose will produce the highest levels of fulfilment, enjoyment and success. They will provide you with solid and well-defined references for making decisions.

Avoid the twin diseases of superficiality and indecision. Your decisions should be a by-product of your life's purpose. Your decision-making ability is not about being better than someone else. It is about you becoming better than you were yesterday, last week, last month and last year.

For ADHDers making decisions can be like playing a pinball machine, with ideas and decisions bouncing all over the place and flashing lights that distract and confuse the process until exhaustion takes over. The brain short circuits and shuts down the executive function facility.

ADHDers tend to say yes to just about everything to keep the dopamine flowing through constant change, novelty and self-induced pressure.

7 KEY ELEMENTS FOR ACTION

Being decisive must become a way of living; without it, you waste precious time and energy.

SUMMARY

- Decision-making is a repeatable process.
- Making better decisions is a learnable skill.
- Your decisions determine your life.
- Better decisions, better life.

ACTIONS

1. Schedule quiet time to think. Achieve a state of physical, mental and emotional calmness.
2. Only work on one decision at a time. Identify the type of decision, employee, resources, financial, sales, strategies, and the size and importance of the decision to justify lengthy consideration or a quick yes or no.
3. Have a crystal-clear vision or outcome for making the decision.
4. Complex decisions may require much smaller but no less important decisions to be made before a great final decision can be reached. Nominate the size of the decision. Is it:

   - Minor – day-to-day decisions that need to be right 25% of the time, e.g. buying a new printer.
   - Major – larger executive function decisions that need to be right 50% of the time, e.g. a new team member.
   - Massive – Large personal or business-critical decisions that need to be right 75% of the time, e.g. whether to bring an investor in or alter your business or career direction.

5. With major and massive decisions, only start working on the decision when you have gathered sufficient, correct information.
6. Take the emotion out of the decision; get it out of your head onto paper or a whiteboard.
7. Make your major decisions based on the highest possibility of success, *not perfection*, and set a timeline to reach a decision.
8. Once the decision is made, don't start overthinking or second-guessing your decision. Take immediate massive action.

Make critical decisions before you have to.

6. COMMITMENT

Commitment starts with a decision. Lots of decisions get made, but that alone doesn't imply commitment.

Many people are capable of starting the process of change, but when the going gets rough, they give up and throw in the towel, often too quickly.

ARE YOU INTERESTED OR COMMITTED?

An important question you must ask yourself is, are you interested or committed to achieving the goal? As John Assaraf from NeuroGym, one of the leading mindset and behaviour experts in the world, explains, if you are interested in achieving the goal, you will do what is convenient. If you are committed, you will do whatever it takes.

Commitment refers to the degree to which you are attached to achieving your goal and your willingness to pay the price. If you aren't 100 per cent committed, you will be unlikely to achieve it.

7 KEY ELEMENTS FOR ACTION

You can have anything you want in life. You just can't have it all at the same time. Some things will have to wait. Are you willing to keep working at it long enough until you succeed?

Once you commit, there's no looking back. You have crossed that line in the sand, that point of no return. Cut away any concept of failure and direct all your thoughts and energy towards achieving your major goals.

When you fully commit to the decision, you start a series of events and other decisions that drastically improve your chances for success.

Your commitment may not guarantee that you achieve everything you want, but it will drastically improve your odds of achieving anything you commit to.

Being committed helps you say no to distractions. It gives you clarity and helps in the decision-making process.

Commitment is what converts a dream into reality. It is finding the time when there is none. It is getting back up one more time when no one is watching.

You must be committed to your goals and visions that you'll defend to the death and put your precious life's time and energy towards.

You must also be prepared to design and endure the processes and changes necessary to achieve your burning desires.

Commitment has to be reinforced and become a daily habit, just like brushing your teeth. Go over your vision board and goals every morning and feel what it's like to have achieved your goal.

You have to build your commitment from within. Don't rely on external factors to give you the strength and power to hold the line when you are all alone facing temptation, and the maniac roommate in your head is telling you that it's alright to skip the cardio and have a beer and chips, it's only once, and no one will know. You will!

I am not saying you have to live like a monk. But it is better if you choose the reward and the time to enjoy it in advance, rather than being overwhelmed by a random desire to eat a tub of ice cream out of frustration or boredom.

> **Example**
>
> *I struggle with moderation; if I eat sh*t I always eat a lot. Just have a couple of sweet biscuits. Yeah, right, I eat the whole packet. When I was drinking, the same applied. The purpose was to get drunk. I could never understand people who would or could only have a couple of beers. I mean, what's the point?*
>
> *I stopped drinking because I knew if I started, I wouldn't just fall off the wagon. I would run the wagon off the road, over a cliff, and completed destroy the wagon and myself.*
>
> *For me, it's easier if I remove the temptations and plan the break-out in advance as much as possible.*

One person with commitment is equal to ninety-nine who are only interested.

SUMMARY

- Understand the difference between being interested and being committed.
- Be 100% committed to your goals.
- Make commitment a daily ritual.
- Be prepared to pay the price.

ACTIONS

1. Commitment is power. It affects your self-belief, confidence and self-esteem. It is the difference between success and failure. Make it a daily ritual to recommit to your goals and dreams.
2. If you are not 100% committed to reaching a specific goal, dump it and find something that you can be 100% committed to over both the short and long term. You need to see the goal and the necessary commitments as a critically important part of your life.
3. Commitment helps you stick to your tasks, as obstacles and challenges appear when life gets in the way. Use your commitment to reinforce the belief that you can carry out the behaviours and tasks necessary to achieve your objective ... *you are enough!*
4. To succeed, start taking action that matches your commitment. Get outside your comfort zone. Be 100% committed, and you will make better, more effective decisions, and that's what it takes to achieve success.

7. HYPER-FOCUS

Focus is imperative to your success.

Without a doubt, your ability to focus on your goals until you achieve them and defeat the ever-present distractions in your daily life is a critical skill to develop and manage.

One of the hardest things will be saying no to the opportunities that show up that are new and exciting. You are looking for a dopamine hit that comes with new and novel thoughts and activities.

Be aware of your wandering mind and bring it back to focus on your goal and the task at hand. Ask yourself, will this thought or action move me closer to or further away from my major goals? And be honest with your answer.

Successful people aren't smarter than you. Rather, they have better systems and processes that help them focus on their area of expertise. They don't multitask.

Your ability to get and stay focused is both your greatest asset and your biggest challenge.

It is more than just a worthwhile habit to cultivate – it's a critical factor in your success or failure. Getting things done is imperative, and focus is the key to getting the 'right' things done.

The distractions that surround you aren't going anywhere, so learning to selectively focus is one of the best things you can do for yourself.

Your ADHD mind can easily focus on something that interests you. It doesn't require a massive effort. By restricting what you focus on, you can use this ability to your advantage to gain maximum benefit from your subconscious mind.

In our age of constant distraction, focus is a major key to your success. You must be fully engaged in the task at hand. Focus will help you find the most direct route to your desired results.

Focus magnifies your mental energy to power through any challenge, just like a magnifying glass does to the sun's rays.

Kick-start yourself into focused action. Just take the first step and build momentum.

Slow down. Be aware of what you need to get done, and concentrate only on those things. Make every action count. Look to create more value instead of just being busy.

Selective focus is consciously choosing the tasks to work on. Use blocks of time to focus solely on one project at a time and remove all distractions and interruptions, mobile, email and people.

Instead of wasting both your time and money, get organised. Have everything you need to work on the selected major task before getting started.

Create an environment in which you're less tempted to get preoccupied with something other than what you're working on.

If possible, change your schedule to align with when you naturally feel more focused.

If your concentration starts to wander, try a short five-minute break. You need time to clear your mind and reset by doing some exercise, taking a quick walk, meditating or simply daydreaming.

Without a break, it's more difficult to stay focused and motivated.

Set rewards, like a coffee or ten minutes on emails, then bring your full attention to one task at a time – no multitasking.

It also means paying attention to your thoughts and recognising when your mind starts drifting. This allows you to manage what you focus on and redirect your thoughts when you slip up.

If important thoughts flash into your mind, quickly write them down, then put them away out of sight for actioning later and get back on task.

A great way to begin doing this is through the 'Pomodoro technique', in which you set a timer and are completely focused on a task for some time, such as fifty minutes straight. Then allow yourself a ten-minute break.

If fifty minutes is a challenge, start with something more manageable, such as thirty minutes, then give yourself a five-minute break. The idea is to make a game of it – challenge yourself to work diligently on your task until the timer goes off, then allow yourself to enjoy whatever distraction you want, but only for an allotted time.

ADHD ADDults

Try different time blocks to see what works best for you. The longer you can stay focused, the more productive you become. Again, develop the habit and keep improving.

After the break, it's back to work again for the next session. You'll be amazed by how much you can get done using this method.

> To maintain a strong focus, limit the amount of conflicting information you absorb. Don't change direction every day as you learn something new that might be worth trying. This will only scatter your focus and slow your progress.

SUMMARY

- Focus will help you find the quickest route to your desired results.
- Magnify your results with directed focus.
- Set predetermined, uninterrupted time blocks.
- Schedule short breaks to recharge.

> The successful person is the average person, with hyper-like focus.

ACTIONS

1. Prepare – When starting a new task, separate the prep work from the actual work and treat them as two distinct stages. Get what you need for the project. Create a checklist if necessary. Have everything you need before you start.

2. Check your environment. Create the best working conditions for your brain by removing all distractions and clutter from your immediate work area. Isolate yourself if possible. Turn off all distractions. If you're working on a computer, close all unnecessary programs and shut off all alerts that could distract you. Silence your phone and put it out of sight.
3. Select a block of time and set a timer to avoid feeling trapped, panicked or overwhelmed. Not your mobile, which has been turned off or put into flight mode. Try somewhere between 30 minutes and an hour to see what works best for your ADHD brain. Once you start, keep going until the timer goes off.
4. Schedule a break. When your alarm goes off, stop whatever you are doing and discipline yourself to take a break. Grab a glass of water, get up and walk around. Do some form of light to moderate exercise. Reward yourself for your efforts.

Example

I always struggled to start something new and outside my area of competence. Once I started, I was reluctant to stop in case I couldn't find that same level of focus, and I could go for three to five hours of hyper-focused intensity.

Unfortunately, sometimes I would continue to work on something at the cost of not doing something else that was vital in a different area that I needed to do within that three- to five-hour time block.

I have disciplined myself to stop when I say I will, and after about three months of retraining my brain, I can now refocus at will 80 per cent of the time.

*Make the ritual of hyper-focusing a habit.
Consistency and repetition are important. Practice
until it becomes second nature. Value progress over
perfection or procrastination.*

8. SELF-MANAGEMENT

No doubt you have taken on different projects and ideas and worked your arse off without getting the results you wanted.

You can be really busy and take massive action, but unless it is the right action, you are just very busy and exhausted, and you end up frustrated and confused.

Why is that? Your ADHD mind tends to struggle with knowing where to start and what steps to take. You have to take some time to plan and then execute the right actions in the right sequence.

Look at your life as a series of projects. Some will be short and straightforward. Other projects will be complex and require the cooperation of many people for a successful outcome.

Start by defining the successful completion of the project and the ideal desired result. Write it down and clarify it on paper. Then, work backwards to the beginning of the project.

- Know exactly what results you want to achieve.
- Find someone else who has achieved a similar goal.
- Identify and write a list of the resources, information, and skills you need to learn or hire.
- Hire experts in the areas outside your interest or expertise.
- Research people who have achieved what you are seeking. Find how they got there and how long it took. Adopt only those traits that apply to your specific goals and dump the rest.

- Buy one or two of the best books ever written on the topic you want to learn about. Then study, implement, monitor your results, and change what isn't working.
- Live it every day, so you get to know it.
- Seek the fastest way to achieve your goal.
- Become a master of repetition.

Do everything with SOUL; people feel soul!

Bring together all the people whose contributions will be necessary for the project's success.

Focus on finding the right people before you start the project. A shared vision is an ideal future picture of success that everyone buys into.

Brainstorm and list every task, function and activity that comes to mind that must be completed, right down to the smallest job.

The more you can break the project down into individual jobs and tasks, the easier it is for you to plan, organise, supervise, delegate, coordinate and get the project successfully finished on time.

What part of the project – that is, what task or activity – determines the speed at which the project can be completed?

The key to crisis anticipation is to think through, in advance, the different delays and setbacks that can knock your project off schedule.

Use meditation to combat unexpected challenges.

To succeed over the longer term, you need to identify the right course of action for you and stick to it while discarding everything else – at least for the time being.

SUMMARY

- Set clearly defined outcomes.
- Find the right people.
- Plan, execute and adjust.
- Life is a never-ending series of projects. Learn to be a great project manager.

ACTIONS

Select a business-, personal- or health-related project then:

1. Define the ideal or perfect result you desire from accomplishing it.
2. Make a list of every ingredient and step you need to take to complete the project to your predetermined standard.
3. Draw up a master plan. Organise every task and activity that needs to be done in order of sequence from first to final jobs.
4. Find and engage the people and resources you will need to complete each task. Seek cooperation from them and discuss the project in detail. Get them to commit to doing their agreed part.
5. Practice crisis anticipation and determine the challenges that could delay the successful completion of the project. Look for solutions *before* the challenges occur.
6. Take 100% responsibility for the completion of ALL the projects that are vital to your future success.
7. STOP overthinking and overplanning. Start and adjust as you go. Continually evaluate your progress and refine your strategies and actions.
8. Master project management by controlling your thoughts and actions.
9. Don't complain or make excuses. Find solutions.

Only through action can knowledge and information become valuable. There are no exceptions.

NOTES

13

YOUR SUCCESS

'Successful people do what unsuccessful people are not willing to do. Don't wish it were easier; wish you were better.'

Jim Rohn

RESULTS OR PROCESS?

I believe your ADHD brain needs both.

Your success is the combined efforts of your beliefs, thoughts and actions, both conscious and subconscious. Some results could come today or tomorrow, maybe six months from now or years later.

With a results-oriented bias, you value performance over the process. Being results-driven, you focus on results, set specific end goals, and then create strategies and action plans to achieve them.

The results-driven mindset has some notable advantages. First of all, because of its focus on results, needs will be addressed as and when they arise. This results focus drives your passions, provides energy, creativity, and by default, leadership.

From your ADHD executive function perspective, your focus is on meeting your goals and objectives; dopamine-releasing performance is valued higher than process.

Your results can teach you about your personal philosophies, attitude, habits and discipline and are like the signposts on a highway.

They are there to keep you on the road to your chosen destination. You may have to take the odd detour or back road to get around unforeseen obstacles. You may even have to change vehicles. However, multiple roads lead to your desired destination.

Instead of resisting it, you have to stay focused on your destination and go with the flow. Keep this in mind when you are evaluating a detour or challenging situation.

When a result fails to happen, don't get caught up in this particular result. Be smart and see past where you are right now. Keep going for what's rightfully yours. You are supremely adaptable and can learn anything.

You are going to have to become a different person if you want to get different results. Recognise the benefit of using failure as a stepping stone to your ultimate success.

You need to regularly check your results to keep on track. If some areas are not up to speed, check what is holding you back. Is it your discipline, your beliefs, or is the goal not that important to you?

Starting is wonderful, but finishing is what matters. Success should be measured by both the external value you gain from your endeavours and the internal benefit you receive from delivering on what you set out to do.

YOUR SUCCESS

WHY RESULTS ARE IMPORTANT

The importance of your results varies considerably. If you are hoping to start a family, your pregnancy test results are very important. The results of the decision to order takeaway from a place you haven't used before, not so much.

Results should be easy to access, a yes or no, but are neither positive nor negative. It is your thinking that makes it so.

Results also allow you to see your failures, so you can learn and improve. Use your results to teach you about your activities, your attitude, your habits, your discipline and your philosophy.

What gets measured gets managed. Your results allow you to see if you are making reasonable progress within a reasonable time.

☺

Results or excuses, your choice.

PROCESS

Even a result that you failed to achieve is still a result that you can feel good about when you use it to improve and grow.

You can also achieve a specific result and think it's not what you thought it would be. Simply accept it, learn from it, and set different goals. It is a journey. Life changes, and there is no finish line.

Enjoy striving to get the results you want, let go of the outcome and be aware of some of the better opportunities that arrive when you don't get the result you expect.

Your results are a means to an end. Any result by itself is just a piece of the jigsaw puzzle that makes up your life. The combination of lots of big and small results, failures and successes over many years, makes up your jigsaw picture.

Monitoring your results helps to hold you accountable for your actions. They make it easy to see how you are doing and see if you need to make adjustments in your processes to move you closer to your desired goals.

Results do matter in that they're something to aim for and something to respond to. It's like a chess match – one move gives you the choices for the next move. Without a challenger, there would be no game. And it's the desire to be in the game, to grow and evolve, which is part of your true nature.

On the downside, focusing solely on results can lead to a narrow perspective. And because your focus is on a very specific result, you might miss out on other opportunities to achieve your desired results faster.

> *ADHDers can get caught up in the process. You can spiral down the rabbit hole of information overload that leads to feeling overwhelmed.*

Your brain is chasing the dopamine that is released when you learn something new and exciting. Your mind gets to be creative, to see lots of possibilities without having to take action to realise them during the process stage.

This can lead to overthinking, or chasing perfection, which becomes chronic procrastination and yields zero results.

Learn to enjoy the process over which you have complete control. Work on finding a balance between the process and results that work for you.

SUMMARY

- Success or excuses, your choice.
- Success is not a limited resource.
- Your ADHD brain naturally values dopamine-releasing results higher than the process.
- All success requires both process and result.
- Your success is caused by your beliefs, thoughts, emotions, behaviours, habits and actions.

ACTIONS

1. All successful people have fears. They don't let fear stop them. Learn to act despite your fears.
2. As long as it is morally and ethically right, do whatever it takes.

    - There will always be challenges. Confront them head-on and deal with them.
    - Success has a price. Know what it is, and be prepared to pay it.
    - Train yourself to become bigger than any problem.
    - Success is holding yourself to a higher personal standard and focusing on the process of continually becoming better.

3. Success is not about what you think or say. It's only about what you do. Start by taking some form of action today and every day towards your ideal life. Think big – start small.
4. Failure is not an option. Never, never, never give up.

NOTES

CONCLUSION

Congratulations! You've just finished the final chapter, and your ADHD brain is spinning with possibilities.

Now picture yourself three years from today ...

Look back to where you were when you first started your journey. By reading and implementing the lessons from this book and taking consistent action, you have created this extraordinary life for yourself.

You have broken free from the chains of your ADHD thinking and are living the life of your dreams. Your ADHD is real and brings its own unique challenges and talents.

ADHD is an explanation but *never* an excuse. You didn't let these four letters or other people define who you think you are, what you are capable of, or prevent you from achieving your goals and dreams.

You have managed your ADHD traits to your advantage. You have learned and evolved into your new identity, the person you were meant to be, by overcoming fear and procrastination.

You are aware of but not ruled by fear. Knowledge plus action is your vaccine for fear.

You have dumped all the ADHD baggage on the ground; you are walking more erect and powerfully towards a brighter future.

You know you are not broken, just different, and have learned to work to your many strengths, delegate and compensate for your lack of interest and skills in other areas. You are living the life you designed in the location and environment of your choice.

You accepted total responsibility for changing your limiting beliefs, your thoughts and actions and have honoured your self-promises to do whatever was required, without complaint through self-discipline and commitment.

Your new and empowering beliefs have helped you gain better control of your thoughts and feelings, so they work for you rather than against you to direct your actions towards your major life goals and dreams.

You've taken consistent action and applied the knowledge from this book, ADHD ADDults.com, and others. You have added your own experiences into the mix and adjusted along the way.

You are fit, happy and healthy from practising self-care over self-indulgence. And you have found creative and constructive ways to get the dopamine your ADHD brain needs for you to perform at your optimum level.

You have tapped into the power of your subconscious mind to find answers, solutions and creative ideas that your intellect couldn't solve. This also allowed you to make better decisions.

You've developed more clarity about your mission and are working on achieving and refining it as you gain more experience and knowledge that reflect your values and priorities.

You have developed your self-management skills by mastering self-doubt and building your self-confidence while managing your energy and investing your time and resources into worthwhile projects.

Awareness has helped you stop overthinking, empowering you to take more decisive action. You established rituals, routines and habits that have provided the structure to keep you on track to achieving your goals and dreams.

You have created this exceptional life of your dreams.

'I learned this, at least, by my experiment: that if one advances confidently in the direction of their dreams, and endeavors to live the life which one has imagined, you will meet with a success unexpected in common hours.'

Henry David Thoreau

CALL TO ACTION

Your personal development is one of the most frustrating, challenging and ultimately rewarding adventures you can embark on.

Your whole life has been about personal development or you would still be sitting in preschool. Now you get to choose the direction and level of your personal development.

Your inner journey will completely alter your life for the better. You will be different because you have different beliefs and different thoughts that lead to different actions and different results. Being different is your strength; use it!

Your success lies within your amazing ADHD mind. Learn to understand how it works.

One of the biggest mistakes I believe you might make when trying to improve your life is one of the simplest. You just don't take action on what you learned from information, blogs or books.

It is better to study one book intensely and apply five to seven action steps that you believe will make the biggest difference in your life than to read ten books and fail to take any life-changing action.

So, please, if you do nothing else, apply what you have learned and take massive action with intent, commitment and perseverance.

Repetition is the formula for change, so continue to go over the information in this book. As you reread it, other ideas and solutions will stand out that you missed before.

> *You can make no greater investment than investing in your personal development.*

WHAT'S NEXT?

Take a couple of days to reflect on what you have learned. Then review the notes you have written and work your way through each chapter in sequence again and complete or refine the action steps in each chapter.

This is to get you started again after going through the process once. Repetition is important ... I encourage you to stop overthinking and start doing more.

Put these proven principles into practice – now. Stop the excuses and the procrastination. This is your one life!

Now is the time to commit and start living life as the person you really want to be, doing what you want to do and having what you want to have.

From now on, commit to stop self-sabotaging yourself. Separate yourself from the mob. Decide to be extraordinary and do whatever it takes.

You have an obligation to yourself and the world to become to best you can be.

Your extraordinary life is waiting. Get cracking.

CONCLUSION

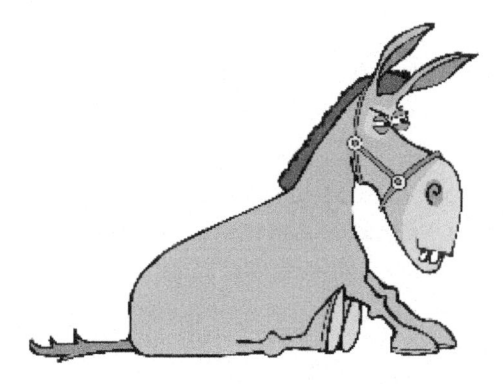

Get off your ass and have a red-hot go!

Hello, Could You Help?

I'd love to hear your opinion about my book.

Your review will help other readers find out whether my book is for them. It will also help me reach more readers by increasing the visibility of my book.

I'd be very grateful if you'd post a short review on Amazon. You can leave your review here (https://www.adhdaddults.com/your-thoughts) … I greatly appreciate your support! Cheers.

References

1. Cortese S, Coghill D. Twenty years of research on attention-deficit/hyperactivity disorder (ADHD): looking back, looking forward. Evid Based Ment Health 2018; 21:173–176

2. *Russell A. Barkley*, Ph.D

3. Del Campo N, Chamberlain SR, Sahakian BJ, Robbins TW. The Roles of Dopamine and Noradrenaline in the Pathophysiology and Treatment of Attention-Deficit/Hyperactivity Disorder. *Biol Psychiatry.* 2011;69(12):e145-157. doi:10.1016/j.biopsych.2011.02.036

4. Stephanie Watson, Executive Editor, Harvard Women's Health Watch July 20, 2021

5. Alison Kravit, Psy.D., AAC January 17, 2022

6. Understanding Positive and Negative Emotion Richard J. Davidson, Ph.D., is the Vilas Professor of Psychology and Psychiatry at the University of Wisconsin-Madison.

7. Fosco WD, Kofler MJ, Groves NB, Chan ESM, Raiker JS. Which "working" components of working memory aren't working in youth with ADHD?. *Journal of Abnormal Child Psychology.* 2020;48(5):647-660. doi:10.1007/s10802-020-00621-y

8. Alan Teo, M.D., M.S., lead author and assistant professor of psychiatry at Oregon Health & Science University,

9. Harvard Medical School

10 Brain Rules by John Medina 1

11 Thomas E. Brown,

12 Simon Laughlin, professor in the department of zoology at Cambridge University

13 G E Tafet[1], V P Idoyaga-Vargas, D P Abulafia, J M Calandria, S S Roffman, A Chiovetta, M Shinitzky

14 Deanne Albon - Be Brain Fit

15 Cowen AS, Keltner D. Self-report captures 27 distinct categories of emotion bridged by continuous gradients. Proc Natl Acad Sci USA. 2017;114(38):E7900-E7909. doi:10.1073/pnas.1702247114

16 Harvard Medical School, Harvard Health Publishing

17 Written by Matthew Thorpe, MD, PhD and Rachael Link, MS, RD — Medically reviewed by Marney A. White, PhD, MS, Psychology — Updated on October 27, 2020

18 WebMD By Stephanie Watson Medically Reviewed by Smitha Bhandari, MD on September 13, 2020

19 CHADD ADHD and disruptive behaviour disorders

20 Science Daily Brain scientists led by Sebastian Haesler (NERF, empowered by IMEC, KU Leuven and VIB) have identified a causal mechanism of how novel stimuli promote learning.

ADHD ADDults Toolbox Index

A

Aaron Beck, 139
abilities, 12, 13, 17, 20, 26, 34, 35, 39, 40, 42, 60, 85, 92, 98, 102, 105, 111, 128, 145
accepted beliefs, 48
action results, 186
action steps, 231, 232
ADDers, 205
ADHD abilities, 13, 20
ADHD ADDults, 1, 5, 165, 230, 237
ADHD ADDults community, 165
ADHD baggage, 229
ADHD brain, 16, 28, 42, 60, 65, 68, 72, 102, 117, 119, 130, 138, 145, 165, 170, 175, 180, 217, 223, 227, 229, 230
ADHD brain structure and clear objectives, 119
ADHD brain's pathways., 117
ADHD challenges, 30, 105
ADHD coach, 165
ADHD coaching, 41
ADHD disability story, 26
ADHD display, 29
ADHD Express, 15
ADHD impacts, 43
ADHD individuality, 15, 123
ADHD individuals, 41
ADHD interests, 122
ADHD mind, 16, 17, 18, 25, 32, 45, 46, 53, 74, 75, 80, 203, 208, 214, 218, 231
ADHD mind dislikes, 75
ADHD mind works, 17, 18
ADHD package, 20
ADHD people, 77
ADHD PFC, 36
ADHD skills, 63, 76
ADHD specialist, 196
ADHD strengths, 18, 31
ADHD support, 43, 196
ADHD support group, 196
ADHD talents, 93, 127
ADHD thinking, 229
ADHD thoughts, 138
ADHD traits, 17, 229
ADHD treatment works, 41
ADHD world, 17
ADHDers, 17, 21, 25, 28, 31, 37, 59, 74, 113, 119, 121, 129, 146, 158, 176, 186, 188, 189, 208, 226

ADHD-limited working memory, 162
Albert Einstein, 69, 119, 145
Amazon, 138, 233
anger, 36, 102, 156, 187
ANTs (automatic negative thoughts), 27, 73
anxiety disorder, 144
approach discipline, 203
Aristotle, 84
associated emotions building, 150
attention and behaviour, 19
automatic negative thinking, 140
automatic negative thought floating, 141
autopilot and start, 60

B

basic emotions, 156, 160
Baumeister, 40
BDNF, 140
behaviour disorder, 19
behaviour experts, 210
behavioural coaching, 41
behaviours and actions cause, 185
belief and fear, 97
beliefs and emotions, 89
beliefs and identity, 81, 88, 150, 174
better decisions, 194, 209, 230
better experience, 73
body armour, 21

body fat, 129, 189
body language, 155
body weight, 28
brain cell formation, 140
brain chemicals, 140
brain chemistry, 59
brain filters, 86
brain fires, 158
brain fog, 196
brain pathways, 34
brain power, 196
brain structure, 119, 133
brain's ability, 28, 184, 195
brain's fear centre, 140
brain's self-management system, 19
brain-derived neurotrophic factor, 140
brainstorming, 66
Brainstorming, 147
building self-confidence, 184
building self-discipline, 202
business-critical decisions, 209

C

career dreams, 106
catastrophic failures, 17
central belief, 91
challenges and benefits of ADHD, 23
Charles Duhigg, 9, 180
chemical issue, 19, 42
chemical variations, 19
chronic procrastination, 75, 226

clean slate, 77
Cognitive scientists, 146
Cognitive-behavioural therapists, 138
comfort zone, 184, 213
common attribute, 25
common attribute of ADHD, 25
Complex decisions, 209
conscious actions, 48, 178
conscious awareness, 105
conscious control, 173
conscious decisions, 55
conscious feelings, 164
conscious mind, 27, 45, 46, 47, 48, 49, 54, 55, 110, 148, 178, 200
conscious thoughts, 27, 48, 110
Consistency and repetition, 218
Consistent progress, 114
constant action, 193
constant distraction, 214
constant torment, 106
core beliefs, 89, 90, 91, 104, 114
core values, 65, 66, 67, 68, 102, 122
creative ADHD, 74
creative mind, 76
creative thinking, 53, 142
creative visualisation process, 71
creativity and imagination, 39
critical decisions, 210
cumulative effect, 184
cycling thoughts, 138

D

daily ritual, 170, 179, 212, 213
daydreaming, 215
decision-making, 34, 35, 76, 91, 102, 205, 208, 209, 211
decisive action, 230
deepest dreams, 106
destructive behaviour, 105, 106
destructive emotion, 157
different' approach, 93
disempowering beliefs, 77
disempowering effect, 32
DNA, 17, 65, 72, 122
doorway to fear, 186
dopamine, 11, 12, 28, 29, 30, 35, 38, 39, 43, 52, 110, 120, 129, 140, 158, 173, 175, 176, 179, 196, 202, 208, 213, 224, 226, 227, 230
dopamine fix, 29
dopamine flow, 52
dopamine level, 196
dopamine release, 30
dopamine reward, 30, 35
dopamine reward system, 30
dopamine rewards, 30, 120, 129
dopamine shortage, 28
dopamine-releasing results, 227
dopamine-seeking behaviours, 179

E

effective decisions, 213
element of thinking and problem-solving, 144

emergency personnel, 29
emotional attachment, 116
emotional awareness, 165
emotional baggage, 90
emotional challenges, 90
emotional cocktail, 155
emotional connections, 41
emotional discomfort, 85
emotional energy, 33, 163, 194
Emotional energy, 194
emotional event, 154
emotional experience, 153, 161
emotional extremes, 102
emotional issue, 188
emotional resilience, 156
emotional states, 154
emotions and actions, 160
emotions and feelings, 36, 82, 83, 154, 165
emotions and feelings drive, 165
Emotions drive, 163
empowering belief system, 110
empowering beliefs, 93, 104, 106, 107, 110, 111, 230
empowering core belief, 116
empowering media, 179
empowering podcasts, 179
energy conservation, 85
energy dip, 196
energy levels, 33, 194, 195, 196
energy management, 31, 34
eurodegenerative diseases, 140
ever-present distractions, 213
evolutionary standpoint, 155
exact experience, 50

executive function, 12, 34, 35, 76, 194, 203, 205, 208, 209, 224
executive function (EF), 34
executive function decisions, 209
external distractions, 180
external visual, 37
extreme cases of fear, 158

F

false beliefs, 82, 85, 88, 89, 90, 92, 93, 99, 103, 106, 150
fear and uncertainty, 143
fear of change, 85
Fear of death, 158
fear of mediocrity and boredom, 133
Fear of snakes, 158
fear response, 158
feelings and emotions, 153
feelings and life, 148
feelings of anxiety, 187
Feelings of dissatisfaction and frustration, 20
feelings of overwhelm, 120, 130
feelings of success, 114
Ferriss
  Tim, 22
financial success, 67, 101
fixed belief system, 97
Fogg
  BJ, 180
food

nutritious, 122, 175
quality nutritional, 43
foods
high-carbohydrate, 196
Ford
Henry, 47
fortune-telling ANT, 139
Freedom of choice, 205
fundamental difference, 153

G

Gandhi
Mahatma, 141
goal-directed actions, 34
Grammy, 22
growth mindset, 26

H

habit
learned, 171
unhealthy, 172
worthwhile, 214
habits
destructive, 173
efficient, 63
negative, 172
Hallowell, 9, 22
health professionals, 42
healthy mindset and discipline, 39
high energy, 26, 29, 71
highest core values, 102
Hof
Wim, 178
home gym, 128

human action, 73
hundred dreams, 197
hundred energy credits, 194
hyperactivity, 26, 235
hyper-focus, 21, 22, 39, 40, 43, 60, 110, 213
hyper-focus abilities, 40
hypersensitive, 24

I

identity
new, 98, 99, 107, 229
old, 98, 99
images and emotions, 71
images and feelings, 47, 50
imaginary problems, 54, 56
imagination and creativity, 68
Improved working memory, 163
Impulse control, 175
impulsive actions, 38
inaction
damage, 186
defeat, 190
inattentive behaviour, 25
individual's experience, 160
infinite universal warehouse, 138
inner voice, 149, 184
inspiring, 43, 77, 112, 165, 178
instant decisions, 155
intelligent action, 183
Intelligent nutrition, 68, 129
intense emotion, 148
interest

shifting, 156
isolation
   physical, 40

J

James
   William, 79
James Clear, 180
Jobs
   Steve, 63
John Assaraf, 9, 210
judgment
   personal, 68
junk food
   , I want to stop eating, 122

K

Kennedy
   Robert F., 62
knowledge overload, 16

L

labelling ANT, 139
lack of awareness, 162
lack of knowledge, 90
lack of self-confidence, 187
lack of willpower, 19, 42
Lama
   Dalai, 53
law of cause and effect, 184, 190
law of discipline, 202
learnable skill, 71, 209
Levine

Adam, 22
Life's challenges, 43
life-changing action, 231
lifestyle
   disciplined, 202
lifestyle choices, 128
limiting beliefs to change, 86
limiting money beliefs, 88
list of empowering beliefs, 111
list of goals, 127
list of goals and dreams, 127
list of negative ANTs, 139
long-term decisions, 36
long-term goals, 32, 35, 38, 39, 175, 202

M

major decisions, 178, 194, 207, 210
Managing thoughts, 35
Mandel
   Howie, 25
Marcus Aurelius, 26
massive action, 117, 184, 193, 210, 218, 231
massive business challenges, 157
massive decisions, 210
master of repetition, 219
Master project management, 220
Maximum brainpower and directed focus, 129
medical personnel, 123

mental energy, 33, 105, 110, 204, 214
Mental energy, 194
mental environments, 35
mental processes, 34
mental self-harm, 106
mental torture, 75
mind conserve energy, 172
mind map, 60
Mind reading, 140
mind spin, 15
mindset
  healthy, 39
  positive, 122, 162
  unstable emotional, 178
misdirected energy, 144
money beliefs
  false, 101
morning rituals, 103, 171
motivation
  lower, 163
  short-term, 60

N

National Science Foundation, 138
natural painkillers, 165
Neeleman
  David, 22
negative ANTs, 139
negative emotion, 116
  strong, 116
negative feelings, 99
negative thought patterns, 140

negative thoughts, 27, 47, 73, 104, 106, 138, 139, 140
Neuroimaging, 19
neurological imbalance, 45
neuroplasticity, 28
neurotransmitters, 140, 195
new belief and identity, 116
new beliefs, 63, 99, 105, 110, 111, 112, 114, 117, 150
new brain cell formation, 140
new habits, 173, 179
new identity deal, 99

O

old beliefs, 97, 112, 122
opposite empowering beliefs, 93
optimum energy, 65, 195
Orfalea
  Paul, 199
organisational skills, 30
outside-the-box thinking, 22
overpowering desire, 88
oxygen pumping, 165

P

pain of discipline, 187
passionate thoughts and emotions, 39
path to freedom, 203
pathways
  effective, 18
Paul Eckman, 156
paying attention, 40, 215
Peale

Norman Vincent, 9, 137
performance
    dopamine-releasing, 224
personal development journey, 110
personal philosophies, 224
personal positioning system, 80
personality traits
    unique, 167
PETs ... positive empowering thoughts, 141
Phelps
    Michael, 22
physical energy, 33
Physical energy, 194
physical health goals, 128, 129
picture
    jigsaw, 226
pictures
    mental, 69, 72
Pomodoro technique, 215
positive affirmations, 116, 140
positive beliefs, 110, 113, 131
positive difference, 68
positive emotions, 148
positive experience, 122
positive headspace, 179
Positive self-belief, 105
positive thoughts, 27, 46, 55, 112, 138
positive, empowering thoughts, 106, 178
powerful emotions, 157
prefrontal cortex, 20, 36
problem-solving abilities
    ,powerful, 145
process
    cognitive, 160
    decision-making, 102, 211
procrastination, 15, 24, 32, 35, 38, 98, 103, 120, 158, 184, 187, 188, 189, 190, 205, 207, 208, 218, 229, 232
procrastination and feelings, 120
Proctor
    Bob, 9, 157
productive activities, 40
project manager, 34, 35, 36, 220
protection
    subconscious, 188
psychological chaos, 15, 20
Purdue University Student Health Centre, 195
pursuit
    disciplined, 68

Q

quality dopamine activities, 43
quicker decisions, 206

R

racing thoughts, 177
Ratey
    John, 22
Reagon
    Bernice Johnson, 43
reality
    new, 200
    physical, 190

physical visual, 147
reality and identity, 98
relationships and self-confidence, 24
renewable energy, 129
repeated actions, 173
resource
  powerful, 69, 70
resources
  brain's, 51
results-oriented bias, 223
Reverse engineer, 130
right decision, 12, 75
Robbins
  Tony, 9, 146
Rohn
  Jim, 9, 62, 187, 197, 207, 223
routines
  daily, 130, 170, 171

S

Sam Altman, 63
self-belief, 100
  True, 105
  unwavering, 103
Self-belief, 100, 103, 105, 107
self-belief and self-confidence, 131
self-beliefs
  false, 107
  Limiting, 104
  subconscious, 102, 107
self-determined actions, 25
self-development, 12, 16, 17, 18, 41, 93, 204
self-development ambitions, 204
self-development minefield, 16
self-esteem and self-confidence, 107, 201
self-evolution, 65
self-fulfilling prophecies, 85
self-help efforts, 41
selfie' beliefs, 103
self-improvement, 16
self-mastery, 201, 203
self-sabotage, 32, 88
self-sabotaging behaviours, 106, 202
simultaneous thoughts, 24
Sir Richard Branson, 22
skills
  creative, 145
sleepwalking, 59
social time, 42
Socrates, 17
solitary success
  single, 184
Spiritual energy, 33, 194
stress drain, 195
Stress-induced emotions, 196
strong emotions, 80
strong emotions and behaviours, 80
structure and rituals, 23
subconscious beliefs, 82, 83, 131
subconscious level, 85, 104, 110, 154
subconscious mind, 46, 47, 48, 49, 50, 54, 55, 56, 71, 81, 86,

114, 115, 117, 148, 178, 214, 230
powerful, 55
subconscious thoughts, 142
success
  project's, 219
successful completion, 218, 220
successful outcome, 79, 85, 218
superconscious mind, 49, 56, 115
sustainable goals, 122
Swift
  Taylor, 23
symptoms of ADHD, 41

T

temporary emotion, 162
term ANTs, 139
thinking processes, 161
Thomas Brown, 159
Thoreau
  Henry David, 9, 18, 231
thought bubbles, 138
thoughts
  'unreal', 72
thoughts and emotions, 53
thoughts and feelings, 45, 109, 159, 167, 230
thoughts flash, 215
time and energy-wasting people, 64
time and money, 215
time blocks
  uninterrupted, 216
time direction, 200
time savers
  real, 199
time schedule, 121
top of mind, 48
Traditional neurotypical methods, 15

U

uncomfortable experience, 188
unconscious belief, 81
unconscious mind, 49
unemotional viewpoint, 109
unique ADHD skills, 63, 76
unique ADHD talents, 93
unique core values, 66
uplifting emotions, 52

V

value
  external, 224
  intrinsic, 102
  true, 199
Value progress, 133, 218
value self-discipline, 67
values
  competing, 67
  deepest, 65
  media, 65
  wrong, 64
Virgin Airlines, 22
visual distractions, 179
Visual processing, 51
visualisation sessions, 71
vocational counselling, 41
volatile feelings, 160

W

wasteful activities, 200
weakness and fear, 201
weeds and ANTs, 73
well-sustained thoughts, 70
work backwards, 218
work challenges, 164
work environment, 31
work ethic, 88
working environment
   normal, 37
working memory, 37, 146, 147, 159, 160, 162, 163, 235
   external visual, 37
   limited, 37, 162
working memory system.
   solid, 37
wrong core beliefs, 91

Z

zero beliefs, 80

Made in the USA
Las Vegas, NV
04 November 2022